THE MICRO-WORKOUT PLAN

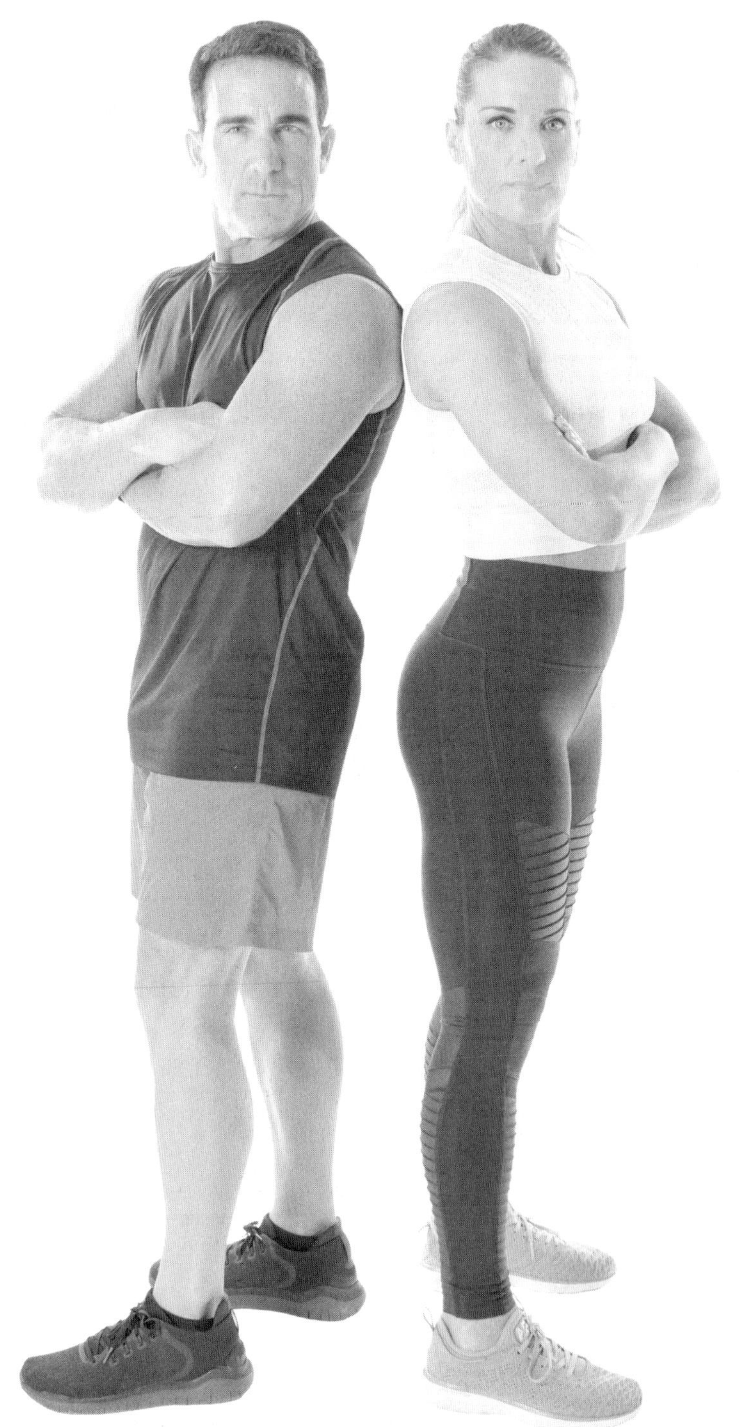

THE MICRO-WORKOUT PLAN

Get the Body You Want without the Gym in 15 Minutes or Less a Day

TOM HOLLAND

FOREWORD BY DENISE AUSTIN

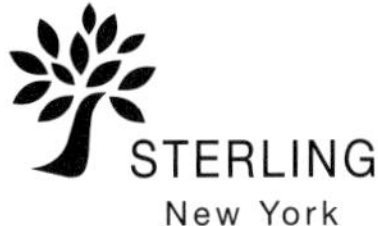

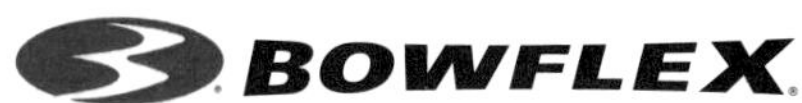

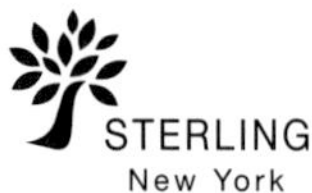

An Imprint of Sterling Publishing Co., Inc.
1166 Avenue of the Americas
New York, NY 10036

ISBN 978-1-4549-3429-5

Distributed in Canada by Sterling Publishing Co., Inc.
c/o Canadian Manda Group, 664 Annette Street
Toronto, Ontario M6S 2C8, Canada
Distributed in the United Kingdom by GMC Distribution Services
Castle Place, 166 High Street, Lewes, East Sussex BN7 1XU, England
Distributed in Australia by NewSouth Books
University of New South Wales, Sydney, NSW 2052, Australia

For information about custom editions, special sales, and premium and corporate purchases, please contact Sterling Special Sales at 800-805-5489 or specialsales@sterlingpublishing.com.

Manufactured in Canada

sterlingpublishing.com

Interior design by Nancy Singer
Cover design by David Ter-Avanesyan
Photographs by Nathaniel Johnston Photography
Illustrations by: Shutterstock.com: Babkina Svetlana, pages x-a, xiv-b, 103, 104, 107, 108, 194-b, 202-a;
Freepik.com: pages x-b, x-c, xiv-a, xiv-d, 102, 105, 109, 110, 194a, 194d, 202b, 202c;
Vecteezy.com: x-d, xiv-c, 106, 111, 194c, 202d

This book is dedicated to
Louise Grace Holland

CONTENTS

FOREWORD

As someone who has spent more than thirty years as a fitness expert, author, and best-selling DVD host, I believe exercise is essential to being healthy, active, and vital at every stage of life.

I know that two of the biggest barriers you have to exercise are the lack of time and feeling uncomfortable in a gym environment. Here's some great news: exercise doesn't have to last an hour to be effective, or even a half hour for that matter. What you need to do is move every day, and all movement counts. You don't have to go to a gym or purchase expensive equipment in order to get in a great workout. Many of my most popular (and most effective) DVD and online workouts utilize bodyweight exercises and dumbbells.

Exercise doesn't have to be complicated or extremely intense to have major benefits. The key is to keep it simple and make it fun. It's about making it part of your day, every day, throughout your day. Cardio workouts will strengthen your heart, improve your mood, and boost your energy so that you feel great. Strength training will help keep you injury-free, allow you to enjoy your recreational activities, and live life to the fullest.

Exercise allows me to be as active as ever. It helps to keep me balanced, stay healthy, and have the energy to be ready for whatever life brings. I continue to enjoy working to help people reach their goals, no matter their age or background, and I know Tom's microworkout plan can help you on your way to a healthier life.

Tom's plan is simple yet effective. It's based on current scientific research, studies he shares throughout the book. It doesn't take a lot of time—the number one barrier to exercise—and you can do the workouts in the privacy of your own home. Shorter workouts work.

As Tom says, you have to stop saying things like "I *only* exercised for fifteen minutes."

Fifteen minutes matter. You matter.

Remember, it's about progress, not perfection.

You can do it!

—Denise Austin

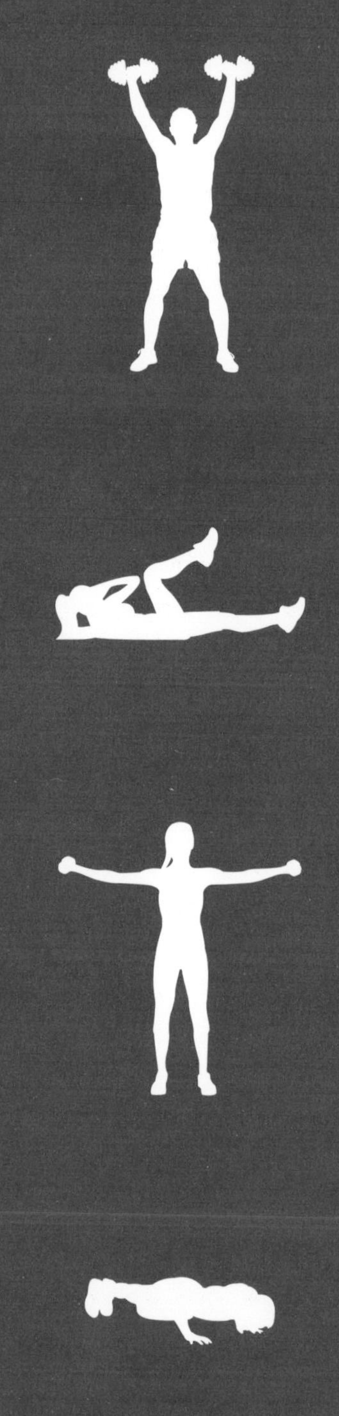

INTRODUCTION

After having spent nearly three decades working in almost every aspect of the fitness industry, I believe the future of exercise is twofold: working out at home, and shorter workouts done throughout the day.

Let's face it: when it comes to exercise, what most people have been doing simply hasn't worked. In fact, it has actually been a colossal failure. Going to the gym for an hour or more (not including the time it takes to get there and back) a few times a week has proved to be an exercise in futility. Pun intended.

Unlike far too many self-proclaimed "experts" in the fitness industry, I am a big believer in facts. Facts matter. Here are two: There are more people with gym memberships than ever before, yet we are more overweight as a society than ever before.

To reiterate: more people are going to the gym, yet more are overweight and obese.

Something is obviously wrong.

Of course, the problem isn't just the gym; it's multifactorial. Diet plays a huge role, as does the decreasing amount of daily activity in modern life. You can go to the gym six times a week, but if you eat unhealthfully and don't get in enough daily activity, you will not see real results. That doesn't mean, however, that the whole exercise-and-gym model isn't inherently flawed. It is.

But this book is not about me bashing gyms. I have spent the better part of my life working in, working out in, and even owning a full-service gym. Gyms serve a purpose. This book is not about quick fixes. It's not about extremes or deprivation or fad exercise programs. None of those approaches work long-term. Many can lead to injury.

As I stated earlier, facts matter. Far too many fitness books are completely devoid of any exercise science whatsoever. In fact, many of the most popular fitness routines contradict the most basic rules of exercise science, which is why they don't work.

So what will this book be about?

Science. Clients. Workouts.

This book is about me telling you the truth, once and for all, when it comes to exercise. Giving you the facts. Imparting knowledge that has come from decades of experience and study and from working with thousands of people. Most importantly, it's about *getting you results*—the greatest results in the shortest amount of time with the least likelihood of injury. Results that will both improve and extend your life.

A few highlights: The book opens with one of my client success stories, because nothing is more powerful or helpful than hearing about how someone actually found real-world success. Chapter 2 is the longest of all the chapters for an extremely good reason—it contains the most common myths and misconceptions, the ones that have been around for years and are keeping you from achieving your goals. I debunk them one by one, with scientific backing, once and for all. Because it's time for you to stop wasting your time. And in chapter 4, I outline the cornerstone of my philosophy, "excessive moderation."

This is a term I came up with that exemplifies my approach, one that has worked for me and my clients. When it comes to exercise, one major mistake people make is that they do a lot, a little bit. They get super-motivated at certain times of the year—New Year's, for instance—and do too much, too soon. As a result, they get injured or burned out, or oftentimes, both. The "secret" is doing a little bit of exercise a lot, rather than a lot of exercise a little bit. The latter is doable and sustainable. That is why five-minute workouts can, and will, change your life. You don't have to take my word for it, either; science tells us so.

It's one of the simplest yet most powerful lessons in life: if you want to achieve something, find someone who has what you want and do what they did to get it. I starting doing this as a teenager by watching, studying, and asking questions of the people in the gym who had the body type I wanted. There is nothing more powerful than real-life examples of people who have achieved their fitness goals. So, in addition to opening the book with the story of my client John, I will end the book by explaining how two other clients beat the odds and not only achieved their fitness goals but exceeded them.

I spend the first part of the book explaining to you *why* you should exercise in moderation, and then I tell you *what* you should do. Thirty micro workouts, each of them just five-minute routines that will absolutely change your life. Hyperbole? Hype? Nope. These are tried-and-true exercises that work. They are one of the primary reasons I am injury-free at the age of fifty, having completed twenty-six Ironman triathlons and more than seventy marathons and ultramarathons around the world. These thirty micro workouts will add both years to your life and life to your years. The one and only catch?

You have to *do* them.

Consistently.

Finally, and most importantly, my ultimate goal with this book is to get you to *believe*. To *believe* that you have control. To *believe* that what you do can make a major impact in the most important aspects of your life. In how you feel. In how you look. In how long you live.

I want you to *believe* that minutes matter.

How do I know? Because I've spent a lifetime studying it. I am living proof. I've taught thousands of people how to achieve this, and now I will show you, too.

—Tom Holland

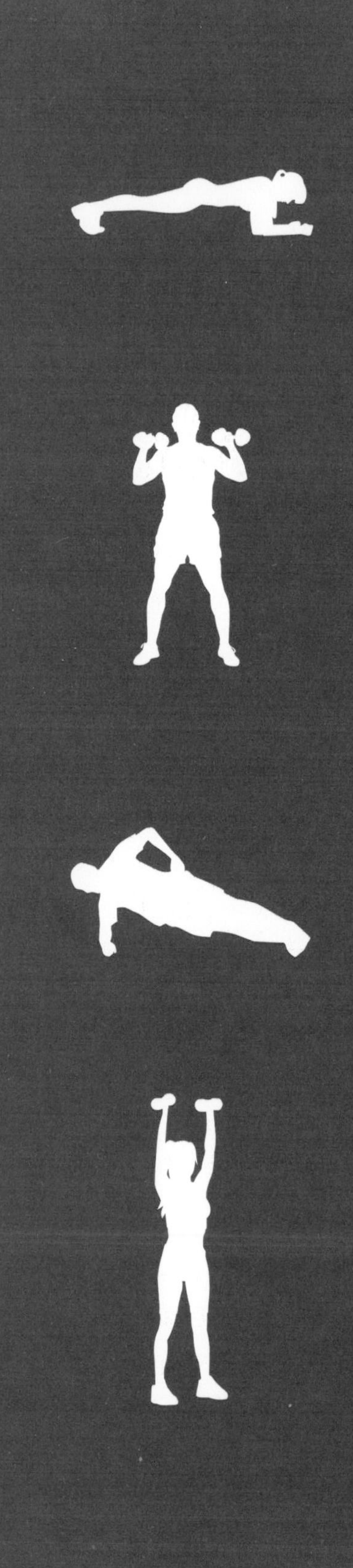

1

BE LIKE BILL

If I were forced to choose one former client out of the thousands I have worked with over the years—one who had achieved the highest level of long-term success with their fitness plan—it would be Bill. He follows the perfect framework of complementary workout routines and doing all of the little things that most people won't. He has been doing it for years, and each and every year he does it even better.

Bill is the personification of "excessive moderation," my term and my philosophy toward exercise, nutrition, and life. It's one of the primary themes of this book, and I break it down fully in chapter 4.

Yet it wasn't always that way for Bill. Not even close. Bill has come a long way. A ridiculously long way. How did he do it? Why has he succeeded when so many others fail? What's his secret?

Bill first found his *why*, and then he embraced excessive moderation without realizing it.

Allow me to back up a little.

Bill started playing tennis as a preteen, and a tennis pro quickly identified his athletic talent. Bill soon began to excel, playing tournaments all over the country and ultimately playing at the highest level in college. He was great at tennis, and he loved it.

After college, Bill went into private equity, doing what so many other young professionals do in their twenties and thirties: working and raising a family. He still loved tennis and played competitively several days a week after work and on the weekends—sometimes more.

In addition to playing competitive tennis, after college Bill took up squash as well, quickly realizing that his athletic ability and years of tennis allowed him to play at a high level in a relatively short amount of time. He had a "split season" of sorts: playing tennis during the warmer months, then going indoors onto the squash courts during the winter. He absolutely loved playing and did so four to five times per week for tennis and two to three times per week for squash. He was also competing in tournaments for both.

Work was great. Leisure time was great. Bill excelled at both. But it wouldn't last.

While Bill was busy building up his private equity business, his body was breaking down. He started experiencing injuries. Lots of them.

First there were the pulled muscles. You name it, Bill strained, sprained, or tore it. Hamstrings. Groin. Calf. Sometimes the injuries would sideline Bill for a day or two. Other times they were more painful and severe, forcing Bill to put down his racquet for weeks, even months.

Then came the surgeries—many of them. Bill had six operations on both his elbows and his knees over a ten-year period, essentially having a joint operated on every two years. There were meniscus tears, severe inflammation, fluid accumulation, and more.

Bill's story up until this point is far from unique. In fact, it's ridiculously common. Many of you reading this book may be doing so because you are *exactly* like Bill. As you have gotten older and continued to participate in your recreational sports and activities, you have experienced numerous aches and pains, injuries, and surgeries. I can't go to a cocktail party or event without people giving me their laundry list of musculoskeletal issues and weekend warrior woes. It has gotten to the point where I remember people not by their names but by their injuries.

"Oh, I remember you. You're the guy who keeps pulling your hamstring while playing soccer on the weekends."

"Good to see you again! How's the tennis elbow coming along?"

I get it. Many of you are injured and frustrated—really frustrated.

When you reach the point of maximum mental frustration and physical pain, you have two choices: stop doing what you enjoyed altogether, or try to fix the problem. Sadly, the vast majority of people ultimately choose the former option. You stop running, skiing, playing golf, or engaging in whatever recreational activity brought you great enjoyment, because your body will no longer allow you to participate.

When you reach the point of maximum mental frustration and physical pain, you have two choices: stop doing what you enjoyed altogether, or try to fix the problem.

You say things like "I used to (fill in the blank), but now I can't because I have (fill in the blank.)"

"I used to run, but now I can't because I have bad knees."

"I used to play pickup basketball, but now I can't because I keep pulling my calf muscle."

"I used to throw the baseball with my son, but now I can't because I have a bad shoulder and it affects my sleep."

"I used to love to play doubles tennis, but now I can't because I have a bad elbow."

You end up choosing another activity, one that most likely doesn't bring you the same amount of pleasure but that your body can tolerate. You feel you have no choice.

Or do you? Have a choice, that is? Is it possible to do the activities you want as you get older, without pain? Without getting injured?

The short answer is yes. You do have a choice.

Bill is 100 percent living proof. He had every reason to stop playing his beloved racquet sports. Or should I say he had every excuse.

Pulled muscles. Extreme back pain. Tendonitis. Multiple surgeries.

So why didn't Bill just give up and stop playing? Why didn't he chalk it up to getting older and just throw in the towel? Many people give up much sooner, even when experiencing significantly less pain and discomfort than Bill did over the years. So why not Bill?

Because Bill found his *why*.

Bill kept going because he was simply unwilling to give up playing his sports. He loved them too much. Tennis and squash brought him an incredible amount of enjoyment and personal satisfaction. He loved the rush of competition and the cascade of feel-good endorphins that came during particularly intense matches. It was his outlet, what he looked forward to after a long, stressful day at work and on the weekends as well. His *why* was simply so strong that he was willing to do anything it took to continue to enjoy it.

While finding your *why* is indeed a crucial element of long-term success with your fitness program, it's not enough in and of itself. Lots of you may have a *why*, yet you gave up on it due to your discomfort and your injuries.

In addition to finding his *why*, Bill embraced one of the most important concepts when it comes to achieving maximum wellness and living your very best life. It's the foundational principle of this entire book: Bill believed he had *control*.

Bill embraced one of the most important concepts when it comes to achieving maximum wellness and living your very best life. It's the foundational principle of this entire book: Bill believed he had *control*.

He didn't believe that his aches, pains, and injuries were inevitable, that they were simply a function of getting older. He believed there were solutions to his problems. He refused to give up, and he refused to give in. He approached his fitness with the same fact-based, methodical, relentless yet patient methodology that he used in the private equity world, one in which he had already achieved tremendous success.

Fast-forward to today: Bill is now in his sixties and is still playing competitive tennis and squash, several times a week for both. He competes in tournaments, frequently beating opponents half his age. As remarkable as it may seem, he is stronger and healthier now than he was in his thirties and forties.

How did Bill manage to come back from so many surgeries and setbacks? What was his secret?

No secret. Bill did the work, and, more importantly, *he gave the work time to work.*

Bill exemplifies every single element of what brings success in fitness and results in optimal health—not one or two but each and every one. Bill's fitness program is the epitome of chapter 4, "Excessive Moderation." He engages in *prehab* so he can avoid rehab, a concept I will discuss in chapter 10. He works on all five components of fitness instead of just one, like most people, the topic of chapter 3. Bill doesn't believe the age-old myths found in chapter 2, and he varies his routine, the subject matter of chapter 7. Bill realizes that short workouts matter (chapter 5) and that his racket sports are a competitive form of interval training, an essential form of exercise, explained in chapter six.

His reward?

Ask Bill, and his first answer will be that he can still do what he loves: play tennis and squash. Yet he won't stop there. He will go on to recite a laundry list of additional positive benefits he has experienced since starting his program, things that are going right instead of what is wrong: He sleeps better, he has more energy for work, he has maintained a healthy weight for years, and, yes, he no longer has the aches, pains, and injuries that he experienced for decades. His good cholesterol is up, his bad cholesterol is down, and his resting heart rate is that of an elite endurance athlete.

If you think you can't be like Bill, you are wrong. Keep reading to find out how.

2

MYTH-BUSTING

There is no better topic for chapter 2 than debunking the most commonly held myths about exercise. These are the myths that have been around forever, the ones that drive people like me absolutely nuts. There are two major problems with every single one of them: First, believing them to be true is one of the major roadblocks to your achieving optimal health. Second, every single one of them has been proven incorrect by science.

Let me say that again, because it bears repeating: all of these myths have been proven wrong. By science. Every. Single. One.

Older generations get a pass. I remember how my ninety-year-old Italian grandmother believed many of them, especially the myth that running is bad for your knees. My parents? They thought about half to be true. Neither generation had the wealth of information we have available to us today—a plethora of studies in exercise science.

What is incredibly unfortunate is that believing these myths today is potentially much more dangerous than it was decades ago. In general, early generations moved more and ate less. What they did eat was more natural and less processed than the food today. That's the bad news.

The great news is that we do have a much clearer picture of exercise science and nutrition, along with a much better understanding of cause and effect when it comes to our health and wellness. We can look to science to tell us exactly what we can control and how we can control it.

So it's time to get rid of these myths, once and for all.

1. YOU CAN'T ESCAPE YOUR GENETICS

This myth is one of the most insidious. It goes straight to the concept of control, or lack thereof. Many people erroneously believe that their health is predetermined by their parents and that it's all hardwired into your DNA—what you will weigh, what diseases you will contract, and how long you will live.

Science says? Wrong.

This is what I consider to be a foundational wellness myth—meaning that if you choose to believe it, the discussion about exercise and nutrition is over. It supersedes all other myths. If you believe this idea to be true, then, along that same line of thinking, there is simply no point in exercising or eating healthy. It won't make a bit of difference. With this idea in mind, living a healthy lifestyle is all just an enormous waste of time. It's out of your hands.

Studies from several important sports medicine journals, and one from the *American Journal of Clinical Nutrition* (item four), support how important strength training and cardiovascular exercise are for changing the trajectory of your overall health:

- The position of the American College of Sports Medicine is that regular exercise can combat the negative effects of a sedentary lifestyle and increase life expectancy by preventing or decreasing the progression of numerous chronic diseases and disabling conditions. Studies also show significant psychological and cognitive benefits from regular exercise participation by older adults. Ideally, an exercise prescription for older adults should include aerobic exercise, muscle strengthening exercises, and flexibility exercises.

- Lifting weights for less than an hour a week may reduce your risk for a heart attack or stroke by 40 to 70 percent; doing more did not yield any additional benefit. The benefits of strength training are also independent of aerobic activities including walking and running.
- Strength training has been shown to have myriad positive health benefits, including assisting in the prevention and management of type 2 diabetes; enhancing cardiovascular health by reducing resting blood pressure, decreasing bad cholesterol (LDL), and increasing good cholesterol (HDL); promoting bone mineral density; reducing low back pain; and easing discomfort associated with arthritis and fibromyalgia. It has also been shown to reverse specific aging factors in skeletal muscle.
- Strength training is an effective way for healthy older people to increase metabolism, decrease body-fat mass, and combat muscle loss, all of which can help with weight management as you age.

Some of you may be familiar with the story of Jim Fixx. He was the author of numerous books, including *The Complete Book of Running* (1977), which sold more than a million copies and helped launch the running boom of the seventies and eighties. He became a running guru of sorts, introducing running as a form of recreational exercise.

Jim was at the forefront of the jogging-as-exercise movement for a few years until tragically, he was found not breathing on the side of a road in Cape Cod at age fifty-two. He had been out running when he suffered a heart attack and passed away.

Many people latch onto stories like Jim Fixx's as proof positive that you can't escape your genetics. They talk about how running and cardiovascular exercise make no difference and how your longevity is out of your control.

Using examples like Jim Fixx is an easy way out, and it's honestly an uninformed example as well. What most people don't know is that Jim had an extensive list of risk factors. His father had a heart attack at thirty-five, which he survived, but ended up passing away at age forty-three. Jim had also been a smoker and overweight, and he'd worked a stressful job for years.

Jim's primary physician stated that Jim had most likely extended his life through exercise and that, had he not taken up running when he did, he would have passed away much younger, just like his father.

I would add that Jim's quality of life was undoubtedly significantly enhanced by his fitness routine. He felt better day in and day out. His losing weight and stopping smoking were also side effects of his exercise. As I will discuss in greater detail in chapter 10, "Prehab vs. Rehab," exercise adds not only years to your life, but also life to your years.

2. RUNNING IS BAD FOR YOUR KNEES

It's simply common sense, right? Running and the associated stress it puts on your knees must be counterproductive. We hear this myth all the time. I can't have a discussion about all the endurance events I have participated in without someone saying, "Yeah, but how are your knees?"

They're great, thanks for asking. No issues whatsoever.

But I'm the *exception* to the rule, right? The pounding that your knees take from running has to be harmful to the health of your knees. Well, not according to science. In fact, what many people believe to be the negative consequences of running are in fact the complete opposite.

It turns out that we were born to run after all. Not only is running not bad for your knees, it actually has numerous *protective* benefits. In fact, runners have a lower incidence of osteoarthritis than nonrunners.

Let me say that again, because it bears repeating, over and over: according to studies, people who pound the pavement have *lower* rates of arthritis in the knees than people who don't run.

The takeaways from numerous studies published in sources ranging from the *European Journal of Applied Physiology* to the *Arthritis Care & Research Journal* of the American College of Rheumatology to the journal *Knee Surgery, Sports Traumatology, Arthroscopy* are conclusive:

- Runners do not have a greater prevalence of knee osteoarthritis than nonrunners.
- A single half-hour session of running has beneficial effects on the knee, including *reducing* inflammation and *lessening* levels of cytokines, a protein that can be a marker of arthritis.
- Running is not associated with increased odds of knee pain and arthritis. In fact, for knee pain, there was a dose-dependent inverse association with running where *runners had less knee pain*. In other words, the more they ran, the less pain they had.
- A multiyear study of almost 75,000 runners found that, contrary to popular belief, running not only doesn't increase the risk of developing osteoarthritis, but these runners were also found to be *less likely* to have arthritis than nonrunners.
- The high-impact forces associated with long-distance running are well tolerated even in marathon beginners and do not lead to clinical relevant cartilage loss.

So running is actually good for your knee joints, not bad. That's pretty amazing. This is an example of a fitness myth that is not only factually incorrect but also the complete opposite of what science tells us.

So how can this be the case? What is it about running that benefits your body?

So often the answers to these types of fitness questions come down to common sense. We can look to Occam's razor, or the philosophic principle that the simplest explanation is most likely to be the correct one.

When it comes to the health of our joints, especially our knees, two factors are crucial.

1. Healthy weight
2. Movement

Runners tend to weigh less than nonrunners. Carrying around excess weight, especially significant weight, places tremendous stress on the knee joints. Think about it: what challenges your knees more, running four miles three times a week or carrying around twenty extra pounds (9 kg) twenty-four hours a day, seven days a week?

I like to break these concepts down a step further by using simple math. Let's say you run nine-minute miles on average and run four miles (6.4 km), three times a week. That comes down to just over 30 minutes per workout, for a total of around 105 minutes per week.

So that's less than two hours out of a 168-hour week. Even if you run four miles every day, twenty-eight miles per week, that's still just over four hours total. This is a small fraction of your time, and most people don't run every day, either.

As I note several times in this book, running burns a lot of calories. It is therefore a great form of exercise when it comes to weight management. Yet one of the reasons running torches so many calories is that it is weight-bearing, which means it is challenging for many people. Add in extra weight and running becomes even more difficult.

When breaking down the efficacy and value of different forms of exercise, I like to start the process by looking at how we evolved as humans. Keeping it simple. Back to Occam's razor. Let's see what nature tells us.

Do you really think that we evolved over thousands of years to sit still for hours on end, staring at a video screen, or were our bodies designed to run through woods and fields, looking for food and shelter?

Personally, I think the answer is pretty obvious.

In addition to runners weighing less and having less stress on their knee joints as a result, the physical act of running is beneficial. Running causes compression in the knee joint, bringing in fluid and nutrients while flushing out metabolic waste substances that cannot be used and are left over by metabolic processes, including nitrogen compounds, CO_2, phosphates, and sulphates.

The problems people have with running are essentially the same problems they have with exercise in general: people do too much, too soon, and there is no balance. If you start slowly, progress intelligently, and engage in cross-training, then running is a healthy, natural form of exercise.

"Runner's knee," also known as chondromalacia patellae and patellofemoral syndrome, is one of the most common forms of knee pain. Often caused by improper tracking of the kneecap due to muscular imbalances and weaknesses, runner's knee can often be remedied through a simple strength-training protocol, including the one found in my lower body strength program (see page 107).

I do triathlons for several reasons, with one of the primary being that it forces me to cross-train. I run a little, bike a little, swim a little, and strength train a little, rather than do just one exclusively.

3. YOU'RE TOO OLD TO START

Not only is this not true according to science, it turns out that when it comes to strength, you can make incredible gains in your sixties, seventies, and beyond. This is especially important when you consider the slips, falls, and broken bones experienced by so many in their later years. The stronger you are, the less likely you are to stumble and, if you do fall, the less severe your injuries are likely to be.

More great news.

Studies published in numerous gerontology and geriatric medicine journals show that:

- Strength training improves physical functioning in older people, increasing functional strength and improving the performance of both simple and complex activities of daily living.
- Older men who engage in strength training for the first time will respond with significant strength gains along with positive cardiovascular and metabolic benefits. Not only can they exercise safely at higher intensities but they will exhibit changes similar to those seen in younger men.
- Healthy older adults can engage safely in higher intensity forms of strength training, which result in significant gains in muscle strength, muscle power, and physical performance. Such improvements could prolong functional independence and improve the quality of life.
- Strength training significantly improves function in older people with osteoarthritis while decreasing pain.
- Strength training reverses certain aspects of cellular aging, making improvements at the molecular level.
- Strength training has significant beneficial effects in the elderly, even those eighty and above, including adding muscle mass and improving neuromuscular function—both of which lead to an improved functional capacity during activities of daily living.

Once again, how do you want to experience your later years? Would you like to be as pain-free as possible? Would you like to be active and participating in all the activities that bring you enjoyment? Or would you rather be like the vast majority of people, dealing with numerous musculoskeletal issues that plague them daily and lead to a decreased quality of life?

The choice is truly yours.

4. STRENGTH TRAINING WILL MAKE YOU BULKY

This myth drives me completely nuts. Crazy, actually.

Bulk is truly a "four-letter word" when it comes to exercise. The fear of putting on too much muscle, of getting too big from strength training, is one of the main reasons women fail to achieve their best and healthiest bodies.

It's not going to happen.

Back when I was a trainer in New York City, I had a new female client complain to me that I had made her legs "huge." We had trained together two times a week for three weeks at that point, which added up to six total sessions of strength training. I wish I were that good.

One unfortunate reason this myth persists is that there are numerous well-known celebrity trainers, male and female alike, who literally make their living from pushing the concept. They play upon this unfounded fear, proselytizing about how you need to avoid certain exercises, such as squats and lunges, like the plague, lest you desire to add some serious size to your thighs. This always makes me laugh, because most people already spend their day squatting and lunging—these are movements commonly performed in daily life. Do you really think adding a few sets of squats to your weekly workout is going to turn you into Quadzilla?

So you are warned to avoid certain specific exercises because they will make you bulky, and you are also instructed to use only light weights when strength training. According to this myth, do the wrong exercises or go too heavy and you will get too big.

Pure unadulterated nonsense.

The so-called fitness experts who espouse this myth would fail the introductory course Exercise Science 101. They don't understand the basic concepts, including the progressive overload principle, which states that you need to "overload" the muscle, both significantly as well as progressively, to build muscle mass.

Muscle hypertrophy, or the increasing of muscle size, won't happen unless the following factors are present:

1. A *significant* stimulus (resistance), one that progresses over time.
2. The presence of anabolic hormones, which stimulate protein synthesis and muscle growth; testosterone is an example of an anabolic hormone. Men can build more muscle than women in large part because they have significantly higher levels of testosterone.
3. A significant volume of training; volume includes the number of times you strength train, the amount of weight you use, the number of repetitions, and the number of sets. To put it into perspective, bodybuilders commonly strength train twice a day, six days a week.

You need all three of these to increase muscle size. Bodyweight exercises like squats and lunges do not qualify as a significant stimulus—you do both of these movements many times a day, seven days a week.

In addition to asking you to eschew certain exercises, proponents of this myth also insist that you use light weights for all exercises and perform a high number of repetitions ("Light" is a relative term and depends on your fitness level as well as the muscle group being worked. The general rule of thumb is that, when performing ten to fifteen repetitions of an exercise, the weight should feel challenging for the last few repetitions.) Once again, they would receive a solid grade of F in exercise science.

Research indicates that performing more than fifteen repetitions with light weights works the *endurance* capabilities of your muscles rather than building significant strength and increasing size. In other words, the weight is simply too light and the repetitions too high to break down the muscle tissue. Yes, you will absolutely get better at performing that movement for longer periods of time without becoming fatigued. If your goal is to build functional strength, increase your lean muscle, and boost your metabolism, however, then you need to increase the weight and lower the repetitions.

A 2016 study in the *American Journal of Cardiology* concluded that body composition is important: those with more muscle mass and less fat mass had the lowest mortality risk compared with other body composition subtypes. Muscle tissue is more "metabolically active" than fat tissue. The more lean muscle you have, the more calories you will burn, twenty-four hours a day, seven days a week. Building lean muscle through strength training is therefore one of the only ways to naturally boost your metabolism.

The Burn

The avoidance of building "bulk" while strength training often results in excessive repetitions with extra-light weights. When it comes to doing strength moves with high repetitions—namely twenty, fifty, a hundred, or more—people often reference "the burn" they feel, believing that it is an obvious indicator of the value of the technique.

Fifty bodyweight squats. One hundred kneeling butt kicks. Yes, it burns. No, it is not building the metabolically powerful lean muscle. The burning sensation does not indicate the value of the exercise from a strength and lean muscle perspective. Doing exercises with twenty repetitions or more works the endurance capabilities of the muscle fibers. If you're running a marathon or doing an Ironman triathlon, that's great. If your goal is to build functional strength and what is commonly referred to as muscle tone, then you need to increase the weight and decrease the number of repetitions.

Indoor Cycling

Fear of becoming bulky also extends into certain exercise modalities as well. I spent many years teaching numerous types of group fitness classes, including indoor cycling. To this day, many women avoid these spin classes, believing they will add inches of muscle to their legs. I've heard more than one woman explain how they had to stop taking indoor cycling because it had made their legs bigger, again often after taking just a few classes per week for a few months.

Although they may truly believe that exercises like squats and classes like indoor cycling packed muscle on their legs, it's simply not the case. It's perception, not reality. The resistance the bike provides is simply not close to enough to build this type of muscle mass. I can only surmise that the increased tightness, firmness, and muscle "pump" in the area, resulting from increased blood flow from the exercise, is perceived as the building of bulk.

If indoor cycling truly built muscle that quickly and easily, bodybuilders would be spinning all day long.

Speaking of resistance, many of these classes focus on super-fast pedaling, what is known in cycling as a "high cadence." The RPMs (revolutions per minute) are often a hundred or more, and to achieve this, very little resistance is used.

I have a friend who was a professional female cyclist and then opened up her own indoor cycling studio. She taught numerous classes daily for many years and was often confronted with the issue of cycling and big legs. Her response?

"I would just point at my legs and laugh. Five thousand revolutions per hour will not build bulk."

Finally, the bikes often also have a weighted wheel, which means even less resistance and effort are needed to keep it spinning once it reaches these high speeds.

The bottom line? Indoor cycling will not make your legs bulky. Eating too much and exercising too little will do that. Indoor cycling is, however, a great way to burn calories, alleviate stress, and strengthen your legs.

Body Types

But what about the female cycling instructor with the muscular legs? Isn't that proof positive that pedaling a bike will bulk you up?

This is a great place to discuss the three genetic human body types: ectomorph, mesomorph, and endomorph. These three somatotypes were originally classified by W. H. Sheldon, an American psychologist.

Ectomorphs are generally tall and thin. Some real-world examples might be runway models or hardgainers—both people who have a hard time gaining muscle. But though building muscle may be a little more challenging, it can be done.

Mesomorphs have a much easier time building muscle. Sprinters and gymnasts are two great examples of this body type. Mesomorphs can build muscle more quickly, achieving greater size and definition, than the other body types. I personally am a mesomorph.

Endomorphs have the body type classically referred to as big boned or larger framed. They tend to be rounder and carry more body fat. Football linemen and powerlifters tend to be of the endomorph body type. Endomorphs can build muscle more easily than ectomorphs and, like all three body types, they can achieve a strong, healthy, balanced body as well.

Here's the skinny on body types: they are genetically predetermined. You cannot switch from one to the other. Want a different body type?

You're going to need new parents. It's encoded in your genetics and hard-wired into your DNA. Yet all three body types can look and feel their best through exercise. All three.

It is generally ectomorphs who worry about becoming too "bulky," and it's not going to happen.

The bottom line is that, regardless of your body type, you want to engage in resistance training, full-body workouts that strengthen you from head to toe. You need to use weight that challenges your muscles. You also want to perform cardiovascular exercise that raises your heart rate, burns calories, and provides numerous other essential health benefits.

Long and Lean Muscle

You hear it all the time: fitness products and programs promise results that include building long, lean muscles. Sometimes they take it one step further, stating that their groundbreaking system will actually lengthen your muscles.

Impossible.

These programs are playing directly into the fear of bulk. They are telling you that you can fool Mother Nature and "change" from one body type to another. They undoubtedly focus on high repetitions and low weight, if any weight at all.

Your muscles have what is known in exercise science as an origin and insertion point. These are the places where they are attached to the bone. The only way to actually lengthen a muscle, therefore, would be to detach one of the ends and move it farther up the bone.

So what about all those long, lean body types in the yoga, Pilates, and barre classes? They walked in the door that way. It's what I refer to as exercise self-selection. People with certain body types often choose certain classes. Show me a group of people waiting to take an exercise class, and I will tell you exactly what that class is. Basketball doesn't make people taller. Tall people choose to play basketball.

5. SQUATS AND LUNGES ARE BAD FOR YOUR KNEES

Even after decades in the fitness industry, it never ceases to amaze me how belief in the top myths is exactly what keeps people from achieving their healthiest bodies. This myth about squats and lunges being bad for your knees is without a doubt one of them.

Let's think about it for a moment: are we not already squatting and lunging all day long, as I said earlier? Bending down to pick something up and getting in and out of chairs are just two examples of daily movements that involve compressive forces on the knee joints—the same types of movements involved in the squat and the lunge.

Yet we still have doctors and others in the fitness industry advising you to stay away from these exercises, especially if you are already experiencing knee pain. So you avoid these strengthening exercises, and as a result the muscles around your knees become weaker and weaker and your pain becomes greater and greater. It's a horrible snowball effect and an all-too-common issue.

The exercise science is simple: the weaker the muscles are around a joint, the more unstable the joint. The more unstable the joint, the more pain you are likely to experience. The goal, therefore, is to do everything possible to ensure that your joints are as stable and strong as they can be.

When it comes to knee joints, squats and lunges are an enormous part of the solution. Once again, you are already doing these movements all day long. That's one of the reasons so many people experience knee discomfort. The weakness and instability leads to increased bone-on-bone contact and associated pain.

The line I often use is that squats and lunges are not bad for you—it's bad squats and bad lunges that are bad for you. You need to progress *appropriately*, beginning with the basics and working your way slowly up to more advanced exercises. You need to perform these exercises with *proper form*. Finally, you need to add the appropriate amount of weight and resistance at the appropriate time.

Proper progression. Proper form. Appropriate amount of weight. When these three rules are followed, squats and lunges are two of the most effective exercises at strengthening the lower body, protecting your joints, and helping to improve your quality of life.

Squats are an effective training exercise for protection against injuries and for strengthening of the lower body, notes a 2013 study published in *Sports Medicine*. Contrary to common myth, if performed accurately, squats do not contribute increased risk of injury to the tissues of the knee joint.

---

6. YOU CAN SPOT-REDUCE

"Get flat abs fast by using our breakthrough Abinator! Just four easy payments of $19.95!"

"Take inches off your hips in no time with the brand-new Miracle-HipMelter!"

Another faulty fitness concept that slick marketers have exploited for decades is the spot-reduction myth. It used to be all the rage in late-night infomercials: you are now bombarded with these same claims in ads on Facebook, Instagram, Pinterest, and more. Print magazines and online websites also often have articles with headlines such as "Tone Your Trouble Spots with This Two-Minute Workout."

Genetically speaking, women tend to carry excess body fat on their hips, while men pack on the pounds in the abdominal region. Both genders attempt to target these "problem areas" with specific exercises in the hope of getting rid of unwanted fat.

Science says? It can't be done.

A 2013 study published in the *Journal of Strength and Conditioning Research*, which examined a group of participants undertaking a resistance-training program on their nondominant legs, concluded that the exercises were effective in reducing fat mass in the upper body and trunk, but not in the leg that was specifically trained.

I have seen the same familiar scene for decades at the gym: women doing endless repetitions on the hip abduction machine while men lie sprawled out on the mats, cranking out hundreds and hundreds of crunches. Both groups could be spending their valuable time so much more effectively. This is one of the top reasons they don't see results from these workouts—they're trying to spot-reduce.

You cannot tell your body to remove body fat from certain areas. Just because you feel the aforementioned burn in a particular region doesn't mean you are slimming or toning that spot.

Your body burns fat in a genetically predetermined manner, one you have no control over.

This is why it's crucial that you engage in strength training sessions that work your *entire* body, not just an area you are not particularly pleased with. Workouts that claim to target areas are flawed from the very start.

Realizing that spot reduction is a myth is essential. This knowledge will keep you from wasting an incredible amount of time and money. It will ensure that you are maximizing your workout time and will put you on track to achieving your best body.

7. YOU CAN CRUNCH YOUR WAY TO A FLAT STOMACH

I thought of leaving this myth out because I just covered the concept in the discussion of spot reduction. The problem is that this myth is far too important not to give it extra attention. Even though men tend to carry more weight around their middle than do women, attaining a flat midsection is a top exercise goal for everyone at the gym.

As I explained previously, you cannot successfully work a specific area of your body to burn away the fat. It just doesn't work that way.

2,000 Crunches

Quick story: when I was just starting out as a trainer in New York City, I began training a young aspiring actor—let's call him Charlie—who was blessed with leading-man movie-star looks. Charlie was starting to land roles on television and in movies, and he wanted to sculpt his physique to better his chances in the business. Even though he was in his early twenties at the time, Charlie was already carrying an extra fifteen pounds around his midsection—weight he desperately wanted to lose.

He had recently read that another actor was doing one thousand crunches per day as part of his workouts. Charlie decided that if one thousand repetitions was good, then two thousand must be that much better. To add to the insanity, not only did Charlie want me to coach him through this crazy core routine—he also insisted that I do it along with him.

Two thousand.

I desperately tried to talk him out of it, sitting him down and explaining the science behind spot reduction. I told him that he would be wasting his time and his money, that he should do cardiovascular exercise to burn calories and do full-body strength training to build metabolically active lean muscle during our sessions. I explained how doing two thousand crunches would probably take a full hour to complete. His response?

"Got it. Thanks for the advice. But I'm going to pay you to do two thousand crunches with me."

So, reluctantly, I designed the program. It consisted of roughly thirty different abdominal exercises, fifty to one hundred repetitions of each. Regular crunches. Bicycle crunches. Reverse crunches. Russian twists. Double crunches. You name it, we did it. Side by side, day after day, week after week.

So how long before Charlie saw his sculpted six-pack? One month? Two?

It never happened.

While Charlie had incredible discipline with our marathon ab workouts, rarely missing a session, his diet needed an incredible amount of work. He loved pizza, beer, and other high-calorie, low-quality comfort foods. He wasn't about to give any of that up.

Also, when I agreed to do these sessions with him, it was with the stipulation that he would do his cardio and strength sessions on his own time. He did get on the treadmill occasionally and do some resistance training, but Charlie was much less consistent with these workouts.

I use Charlie as an extreme, real-world example of how it doesn't matter how many ab exercises you do or how frequently you do them; you simply cannot crunch your way to a flat stomach.

Everyone has rectus abdominus muscles, commonly known as a six-pack. The problem is that, for many people, these muscles are covered with a layer of fat. Another way of putting it is that everyone has a six-pack, but for some people it's just farther back in the fridge.

This doesn't mean that you shouldn't do abdominal exercises or that they are a waste of time. They are not. You simply need to be judicious with the time you devote to them and what exercises you choose. First and foremost, having a strong midsection is essential to your body performing optimally. It helps prevent issues like back pain. It improves your ability to handle the tasks of daily living and will positively impact whatever recreational sports you choose to participate in.

If there is one region of the body that truly calls for a five-minute workout, it's your abs. Five minutes of focused core work done consistently will reap incredible benefits. Spend much more time than that and you are taking time away from burning calories or building lean muscle.

More to come on these specific workouts later.

8. CARDIO WORKOUTS SHOULD BE AN HOUR

Says who, exactly? Did you ever stop to wonder why people go to the gym with the specific goal of doing sixty minutes of continuous cardiovascular exercise? What's so special about an hour of cardio?

According to science, not much.

There is nothing "magical" about exercising for an hour. Sure, the longer you exercise, the more calories you burn. But does a cardio session have to be long to confer benefits? Is it a waste of time to walk on the treadmill for just thirty minutes? What about doing the elliptical for only ten minutes?

Just and *Only*

When it comes to doing cardio, you need to take the words *just* and *only* out of your vocabulary. Permanently.

"I only walked a mile today."

"I could just do fifteen minutes on the elliptical this morning."

Every minute counts. There is no amount of exercise that is "too little." It all adds up.

Studies show that three ten-minute bouts of exercise are just as beneficial as one continuous thirty-minute session. In other words, you can break up your exercise, doing shorter sessions throughout your day.

This is incredible news. You can do five minutes of stretching in the morning, go for a five-minute walk at lunch, and do five minutes of core exercises in front of the TV at night. That's doable, that's sustainable, and that works.

You can do five minutes of stretching in the morning, go for a five-minute walk at lunch, and do five minutes of core exercises in front of the TV at night. That's doable, that's sustainable, and that works.

I have been doing these "micro" workouts myself since I was a teenager, when I began doing push-ups and abdominal exercises throughout the day, wherever and whenever I had a few free minutes. I completely transformed my upper body with these five-minute workouts in a relatively short amount of time.

You know why the hour-long workout myth exists, in my opinion? It goes back to working out at the gym. If you are going to pay the money for a gym membership, invest the time it takes to get there, go into the locker room and get dressed, and then shower when you are finished, a twenty-minute workout doesn't make much sense. A five-minute session? That would be pure lunacy.

Also, group fitness classes have historically been an hour long. Boot camp classes, group cycling, yoga—but even that's starting to change, with many classes now lasting only forty-five minutes.

"I Don't Have the Time to Exercise"

The number one reason most people cite for failing to exercise is lack of time. When someone says this, what they're really saying is *"I don't have the time it takes to go to the gym and then do an hour-long workout."*

Well, you don't have to do either one. You can get your exercise in outside the gym, and your workouts can be five minutes long.

Not "just" five minutes long. Five minutes long.

Can you still exercise for an hour if you want to? Of course you can. You just don't have to.

What matters most is what you will hear me repeat over and over throughout this book. It's all about consistency.

9. YOU NEED TO GO TO THE GYM TO WORK OUT

The gym, as we know it, is dead.

I have to admit, I get a great deal of pleasure when I make that statement. As I said in the introduction, this comes from a person who has spent the better part of his life in the gym. Heck, I even owned a gym for a short time, against my better judgment. So why the negative outlook on gyms?

Because the traditional gym model is to get you to sign up, then go the heck away. Why do you think there are so many gym memberships now that cost so little? Because gym owners have found that sweet spot, that magic number that yo're willing to have charged to your credit card month after month without feeling guilty for going infrequently, if at all. (It's around $10, by the way.)

It's a pure numbers game—the LPHV model. Low price, high volume.

The goal of gym owners is to sign up as many members as possible, then sit back and literally bank on the fact that more than 60 percent will stop coming after just a few months of working out. Those members' credit cards, however, will continue to be charged. Gyms simply couldn't make a profit by charging so little if the number of paying members weren't so high. Yet, the percentage that shows up on a regular basis is extremely low.

If just 10 percent of the membership of most gym chains showed up at the same time, there would be pure chaos.

Gyms aren't going away, mind you. They will always be around. They still serve a purpose. The analogy I like to use, however, is that of Netflix and movie theaters: you still like to go to the movies every now and again, enjoying that special, shared experience with others. But thanks to advances in technology like Netflix and Amazon Prime, you will watch many more movies in the privacy of your own home than you will in a traditional theater.

It's exactly the same with exercise. You can go to the gym if you want, when you want, but you don't have to. You can get the same experience, on demand, in your own home. Just as you had to go to the movies to see the latest release years ago, you had to go to a fitness facility to have access to the equipment and the instructors.

Here are the reasons why the gym as we know it is dead and why you no longer need to go to one to get a great workout.

Home Fitness Equipment

No matter what type of cardio or strength workout you enjoy, there are now great machines you can use at home. The options are better and more diverse than ever before, costs have come down significantly in the past few decades, the machines themselves are more effective, and you don't need a large amount of space to put together a great home gym. No room for a large piece of equipment? That's fine—handheld weights will do the trick.

The Internet

Gyms used to be one of the primary places where you could seek out fitness information, whether from the gym owners themselves, the trainers, the group fitness instructors, or even other members. Now, thanks to the internet, all of these questions are right at your fingertips and can be answered at a moment's notice. For free.

Want twenty different exercises to work your abs? Need to know how to perform a squat correctly? Looking for a "Ten-Minute Bikini Body Bodyweight Workout"? Are you bored silly just walking on your treadmill and need some new ideas on how to mix it up? No problem. There are literally thousands of articles and videos on these topics to choose from online.

Content is crucial to both education and motivation. You need an exercise plan, and you need to know how to perform it correctly. Now, thanks to the internet, you can get both in the privacy of your own home.

Fitness Technology

We are living in one of the most incredible times in health and wellness thanks to the explosion in fitness technology. You name it, you can track it: steps walked, stairs climbed, distance traveled, body fat percentage, hydration, sleep quality, exercise recovery, and much more. You can do all this with the instrument of your choosing: your phone, a wrist-based device, a ring, even specially made "smart" clothing.

Goodbye to the days of exercise tapes and DVDs—you now have access to nearly every imaginable form of exercise routine from the instructor of your choosing, on demand. You can stream live classes to your device or bike and run with others around the world on virtual courses, and there is even artificial intelligence that will help you maximize your results by personalizing your workouts to your specific fitness level and goals.

Simply amazing. Mind-boggling, actually. Remember when you had to go to the gym to have your body fat checked? With calipers?

10. IF I STOP WORKING OUT, I WILL LOSE ALL THE BENEFITS I GAINED

This final myth is one that, like so many of the others, serves to keep you from starting an exercise plan in the first place. I completely understand. It's sound logic, actually. Why would you possibly put in all this hard work, investing significant time and money, when it could all be for nothing if you stop doing it, even for a short period of time? Especially when it's something that you probably don't even enjoy in the first place?

Most people realize correctly that they will inevitably take time off from their program because of work issues, family matters, or some other reason. It's not a matter of *if* you will take a break from exercise but *when*. With this in mind, knowing that you will be less than perfect with your routine, you don't want to waste your time.

Let your heart rest easy: it's just not true.

First of all, what exactly would you lose when you take time off from exercise? I love when people make overarching vague statements like "You know, if you stop exercising for just a few months, it's like you never started at all."

I'm living proof that this comment is, as my dad would say, "a load of malarkey." I have taken dozens of hiatuses from exercise since I first started doing push-ups at age fourteen. Did I revert back to my original fitness level each time? Not a chance.

In fact, I have personally experienced the exact opposite of what this myth portends. When I started competing in endurance races, I would lose weight before each race, which included muscle as well as body fat. I would completely stop my strength training workouts that focused on putting on muscle. No more push-ups, dumbbell chest presses, and bicep curls. Yet, even as I got older, I found it increasingly *difficult* to lose this muscle mass, even when I stopped working out. It would take longer and longer to lose lean muscle.

So what happened when the race was over and I resumed my muscle-building workouts? I would gain the lean muscle back in a matter of weeks.

In fact, people would often remark about how quickly I would regain my muscle. I even surprised myself.

I realize that we are all different genetically and that most people don't exercise like I do. That doesn't change the fact, however, that my personal experience illustrates the myth to be patently false.

So what will the effects be when *you* take time off from your exercise program? Will you in fact lose anything at all? If so, what, exactly?

Of course you will lose some fitness. If you are doing cardio and strength workouts and stop for a period, you will see declines in your strength and cardio. When you resume your training, you won't be able to lift as much. Your cardio workouts will most likely feel harder, and you won't be able to hold the same intensity or duration as you did before.

But have no fear—the fitness you earned before you took time off will indeed return. It will not take you as long to regain it as it did for you to achieve it in the first place. We call this *muscle memory* in the world of fitness. Essentially, the longer you've been exercising, the more quickly you will regain what you've lost after eschewing exercise for a while.

The longer you've been exercising, the more quickly you will regain what you've lost after eschewing exercise for a while.

If it were in fact true that you could lose all the fitness gains you made after taking time off, very few people would be in good shape. Regardless of what you see on Instagram, no one is perfect, and life has a funny way of throwing roadblocks in the way of your best fitness intentions. Sickness, injury, work problems, family issues—all of these and more will constantly challenge you to stick to your program.

In fact, periodically taking time off from exercise will actually *help* you reach your goals. That's what they call *periodization* in exercise science. Periodization is the progressive cycling of a training program, mixing up intensity, volume, structure, and periods of rest.

Why do you think professional athletes have an off-season?

This doesn't mean you should stop exercising altogether for months on end. But taking time off happens and won't result in all your hard work being in vain.

NO MORE BELIEVING THE MYTHS

So there you have it. All the top fitness myths laid to rest, once and for all. It should all come as great news, because the main takeaway is that you have the information and ability to drastically change and extend your life.

Now it's time to get to work. We begin by defining what "fitness" actually is through an examination of its five components.

3

THE 5 COMPONENTS OF FITNESS

You might be surprised to learn that in the world of exercise science, there are five distinct components of fitness. Five. If I asked ten people what each of them were, nine out of ten wouldn't have any idea, and one might be able to come close to a few by guessing. Do you know what these five components are?

The fact that the vast majority of people can't name these five components is obviously a problem. How can you achieve your best self if you don't even know what you need to do to achieve it? You can't reach your destination if you don't have directions for how to get there.

Add to this lack of knowledge the never-ending amount of bad information circulating today, and you are really in trouble. Social media, and the internet in general, is overrun with videos by questionable self-proclaimed fitness experts and iconoclastic clickbait articles telling you that you only need to do one of these components and that the others are a complete waste of your time.

Some will even ridiculously tell you that one of these components is the *very reason* you are overweight.

More on this later.

True health and wellness come from implementing all of these five components consistently; yet most people generally focus on just one. That one component is usually the activity that comes easiest to you, the form of exercise you enjoy the most, and the one that favors your genetics. It's basic human nature and goes back to the previous chapter's discussion about self-selection and the types of exercise people ultimately choose. Ultramarathoners aren't skinny simply because they run long distances; they choose to run long distances because they are skinny. Basketball players aren't tall from playing basketball; they choose that sport because it favors their genetics.

Running, swimming, biking, yoga—it doesn't matter how healthy the mode of exercise is or how frequently you do it; if you engage in only one particular form, problems will arise. In fact, the *more* you engage in just one form of exercise, the *less* healthy it can end up being. When you use the same muscles in the same way, over and over again, you are more likely to experience overuse injuries, muscular imbalances, and pain.

Sound familiar?

So what exactly are the five components of fitness?

1. **Muscular Strength:** The maximal force your muscles can generate (or, in layman's terms, how much you can lift)
2. **Muscular Endurance:** Your muscles' ability to contract repeatedly for an extended amount of time
3. **Cardiovascular Endurance:** The ability of your heart, lungs, and circulatory system to sustain prolonged aerobic activity
4. **Body Composition:** In exercise science terms, *body composition* refers to the amount of body fat you have in relation to the amount of lean tissue, which, for most people, would mean muscle tissue but also includes your bones and internal organs. This is your fat-to-muscle ratio,

which is obviously an aesthetic component but can also be measured at home with body fat scales and in a laboratory setting with more sophisticated equipment.

5. **Flexibility:** The ability of your joints to move freely through their natural range of motion

As I stated earlier, most people who exercise focus on just one of these components—the one they enjoy the most and are genetically built to do. Walk into any gym and you will see every one of these self-selecting types represented:

MUSCULAR STRENGTH: These are the people packing as many plates as possible on the barbell, leg press machine, and back row and who are completely focused on setting PRs (personal records) for the sheer amount of weight they can lift. This subset generally performs cardiovascular exercise sparingly, if at all, for fear of losing muscle and strength. Cardio is primarily utilized as a warm-up and is rarely done above an easy intensity or for long durations. Weight belts, hand chalk, and loud grunting are typically part of the muscular-strength lifestyle.

MUSCULAR ENDURANCE: This group lives by the AMRAP acronym, performing *as many reps as possible* of exercises in a previously specified amount of time. Burpees, air squats, and box jumps are all common exercises performed by those whose primary goal is not how much weight they can lift but how many times they can do it. Both the muscular strength and the muscular endurance groups are focused on numbers but for completely different reasons.

CARDIOVASCULAR ENDURANCE: There used to be a woman at my gym who ran eight miles a day, every day, on the treadmill. Same speed and same workout, every day. She wasn't training for a race, either. It was simply her sole chosen form of exercise. Marathon runners, recreational swimmers, steady-state elliptical users, walkers—cardiovascular endurance is one of the most popular of the five components of fitness.

BODY COMPOSITION: Those who focus on body composition may do so for more nuanced reasons than those who pursue muscular endurance or strength. One reason might be a concern with outward appearances. There are also those who live at the extremes in terms of body composition, from the massive bodybuilder to the gaunt ultramarathoner. Genetics and diet are the primary factors behind body composition, with exercise coming in a distant third in order of importance, which can be problematic when it comes to true health.

FLEXIBILITY: Arguably the smallest of the five component groups, the main goal is to maximize flexibility. This group can include practitioners of yoga, Pilates, and other similar disciplines.

We all know people like those described above and on page 35. If you are someone who already exercises regularly, there's a good chance that *you* fit into one of these categories. Do not take it as a criticism. This is one of the very reasons why you are reading this book: to learn how to take your fitness plan to the next level. To maximize your time and efforts. To minimize your chance of injury while maximizing your results.

So the goal is to start to implement and engage in all five components of fitness. I often say that I could go to any of the dozens of gyms where I used to work many years ago—I would see the same people doing the same exercises and, yes, looking exactly the same. Like the Bill Murray movie where every day was exactly the same, it's Groundhog Day at the gym.

So if you are just starting an exercise plan for the first time, congratulations. Focus on slowly implementing all five components of fitness. If you are already working out, perhaps even for many years, I want you to step back and take an *honest* assessment of your current program. Which of the five components are you doing, and which are you avoiding?

Breaking it down a little further, there are those people who focus primarily on strength, those who spend the majority of their exercise time doing cardio, and those who are skinny thanks to genetics and diet yet rarely exercise.

The strength-only group would have a difficult time running just a few miles. The cardio-focused group would struggle to do a set of good push-ups. The skinny-without-exercise group may be preferred on fashion runways, but they often lack both functional strength and cardiorespiratory fitness.

When it comes to flexibility? The majority of people in all three groups often falls far short.

The goal is for you to incorporate all five components of fitness into your exercise routine.

Remember my client Bill from chapter 1? He is thriving in his sixties because he consistently incorporates all five components into his fitness routine. Twice a week he strength trains, focusing on a mix of muscular strength and muscular endurance. Once a week he does Pilates, a phenomenal way to improve flexibility. Three times a week or more he plays racquet sports, one of the best forms of cardiovascular exercise when it comes to both cardiovascular fitness and longevity. Bill stretches in his home gym after each tennis and squash workout as well.

There are an infinite number of ways in which you can implement the five components in your own plan.

Lastly, he also eats a healthy, well-balanced diet, though it's nothing fancy and nothing extreme. He has maintained a low body-fat percentage and healthy weight for years now.

That's how Bill does it, but there are an infinite number of ways in which you can implement the five components in your own plan. I want you to understand, however, that Bill doesn't follow any trends or torture himself with any fad diets. He doesn't do extreme workouts or complicated exercises. He does the basics while covering all five of the fitness components *consistently*.

The basics done consistently and with variety. This is a perfect time to continue the discussion of one of my favorite topics: excessive moderation.

4

EXCESSIVE MODERATION

One of the major flaws of the common, current approach to exercise is that it is about extremes. It seems that the solutions being sold lie at either end of the spectrum: either way too much exercise, or way too little. It has been that way since the beginning of time. People first want the quick fix, and when that doesn't work, they swing too far in the other direction, doing too much—or vice versa.

Neither approach works. Doing too little yields few to no results, and doing too much can result in injury or burnout—or both. So if doing too much or too little isn't the answer, then what is? Wouldn't it stand to reason that it lies somewhere in between? And if moderation is the solution, why isn't it portrayed in the media?

It's actually quite simple: doing too much sells. Doing too much is exciting. Years ago I was actually in a commercial for one of the best-selling extreme exercise programs, doing nonstop jumping lunges and pop squats for hours on end. I nearly blacked out.

Slow and steady? That's an exponentially harder philosophy to get people to buy and to buy into. Slow and steady isn't sexy. It doesn't sell when it comes to exercise programs.

Until now.

It's time to stop the insanity. It's time to stop wasting your valuable time and your hard-earned money. It's time to get results instead of getting injured.

It's time for excessive moderation.

As I said earlier, *excessive moderation* is my overarching philosophy, one that, in just two words, completely encapsulates my approach toward fitness. Instead of doing a lot of exercise a little bit, do a little bit a lot.

Like five minutes, several times a day.

Unlike extremes, excessive moderation works long-term. It's doable, and it's sustainable. It's like "Goldilocks and the Three Bears": not too much, not too little—it's just right. Excessive moderation will change your life without changing your life. It's the long-term solution: small, manageable, meaningful changes made over time.

Circuit-training workouts are a valid alternative to conventional strength training, even though they take less time and can be performed at lower intensities. The journal *Ageing Research Reviews* found that these quicker, less-intense workouts may also be more enjoyable and that people are more likely to continue to do them long-term. Additional studies show that:

- Strength training just twice per week significantly improves insulin sensitivity and fasting blood sugar while decreasing abdominal fat in older men with type 2 diabetes.
- Just one strength training session can have positive effects on sleep.

The vast majority of people I talk to say some version of the same thing: *"Tom, I don't want to do an Ironman, run a marathon, or get a six-pack: I just want to look better, feel better, and be healthier. I want to lose a few pounds, fix a few nagging injuries, and be able to enjoy my recreational activities."*

As I stated at the beginning of this book, my main job is to get you the greatest results in the shortest amount of time with the least chance of injury. When your fitness goals are meant to essentially improve your quality of life, why would you possibly want to waste your time doing more than you need to while risking getting hurt in the process?

For excessive moderation to work, it must possess three essential components. It cannot and will not work without all three of them. The primary reason most exercise programs fail is because they lack one—if not all—of them.

Quality. Intensity. Consistency.

QUALITY

Quality refers to both the type of exercises selected and to the way each and every exercise is performed. You need to pick the right exercises at the right time, and then you need to do them with proper form. It may sound overly simplistic, but it isn't. If people were getting this right, we would have many more fit people with far fewer injuries. Picking the right exercises refers to both strength training as well as modes of cardiovascular exercise.

Too many workout programs are doomed from the very start because of improper exercise selection. It often goes back to the extremes, with exercises and workouts chosen where the risks far exceed the rewards. Another fad workout pops up, one that promises a "new" and "groundbreaking" program. It incorporates advanced moves and high-intensity workouts that are too advanced for but a select few. Blame uneducated and inexperienced instructors along with the ego of the participants—a recipe for disaster when it comes to exercise.

One reason these extreme workouts sustain popularity is that people don't necessarily experience the injury during the high-risk workout itself but rather when doing something innocuous afterward. Make no mistake about it: the workout is where the damage was done, yet it is seldom blamed as being the root cause of the injury. The unfortunate individual performs advanced moves with poor form for several weeks or months on end and then bends over to pick up a dropped toothbrush, throws out their lower back, and experiences significant pain and discomfort.

One reason these extreme workouts sustain popularity is that people don't necessarily experience the injury during the high-risk workout itself but rather when doing something innocuous afterward.

It's similar to bending a paper clip. You have to bend it back and forth dozens and dozens of times before it ultimately breaks. But it's clear—the repetitive stress caused it to fail.

Finally, once the correct exercises have been chosen, they need to be performed correctly. This means several things.

First, the movement itself must be executed with correct form. Once again, this sounds extremely simple, but the vast majority of people I see doing the most basic exercises in the gym are doing them incorrectly. Squats, planks, push-ups—you name it, they are being done with poor form. Poor form leads to both decreased results and to increased chance of injury. Sound familiar? Not getting the results you want or getting hurt—or both. That pretty much describes the outcome of most people's exercise programs.

Second, you need to choose the correct amount of weight, if any, as well as the correct number of repetitions. It may sound like a gross generalization, but men tend to lift weights that are too heavy (blame ego), and women tend to lift weights that are too light (blame a fear of bulking up). Both strategies are ineffective at best and potentially injurious at worst.

So how much weight should you lift, and how many repetitions should you perform? These determinations depend on your fitness level and goals, and, contrary to many of the articles you may have read, there is scientific reasoning in the answer. I will discuss these exercise science principles and go into much greater depth on the best techniques in chapter 9, "The Fountain of Youth" and chapter 11, "Focus on the Negative."

INTENSITY

In the last few years, the exercise pendulum has swung over to the side of "too much"—way over. These extremes can be found in both the popular approaches to strength training as well as in the popular methods of cardiovascular exercise. People are doing too much too soon, and many are becoming injured in the process. While I do consider it to be extremely good news that more and more people are willing to push themselves when it comes to exercise, extra effort has to be exerted in an intelligent and, yes, *scientific* manner.

There is a method to the madness.

Unfortunately, the "too little" approach still exists as well, and will most likely be around until the end of time. As Sigmund Freud stated in his pleasure principle, human beings seek pleasure and avoid pain. If you see a product or program that promises spectacular results with minimal to no effort in just three easy payments of $19.95, purchasing it would be human nature. Getting more by doing less is an extremely effective approach when it comes to selling exercise.

Yet, in the end, it's only effective at enriching the person advertising the program. It's a waste of time and money for the person following it.

So when it comes to intensity, excessive moderation means doing a wide variety of exercise in small increments—aka mixing it up. Some days you might do low-intensity work, and other days you might do high-intensity. When it comes to cardiovascular exercise, most people tend to spend almost all their time in the "gray zone."

When it comes to cardiovascular exercise, most people tend to spend almost all their time in the "gray zone." . . . an area of area where the effort exerted is not really hard, but also not really easy.

What's the gray zone? An area of exercise where the effort exerted is not really hard, but also not really easy. Over time, staying in this gray zone is not a really effective means of achieving your goals.

Just take a look around any gym at the people doing cardio. Treadmills, ellipticals, stationary bikes, you name it—most are exercising in the gray zone all the time. Is there value to working out at this intensity? Sure; it will improve basic cardiovascular function. When it comes to truly maximizing your time and results, however, including losing excess weight and making big improvements in your fitness and well-being, then only by mixing up your intensities will you achieve that and more.

CONSISTENCY

It should come as no surprise that if there is one common denominator in the programs of people who experience long-term success in exercise, it's consistency. When you do something repeatedly over an extended period of time, you tend to get better at it. You achieve results. It's common sense.

Excessive moderation works because it solves the number one problem people have with exercise: time. Or lack thereof.

Most people aren't consistent with exercise because they have been told they have to exercise for long, continuous periods and that they must do it at a gym. Neither of these statements are true (as I explained in previous chapters), which should come as absolutely incredible news.

It's extremely difficult to be consistent with an exercise program when the aforementioned is the supposed formula. An hour-long workout at a gym takes generally ninety minutes to two hours out of your day when you factor in travel time, changing clothes, showering, and so on. That's a heck of a lot of time out of most people's day or week.

In the end, exercise ultimately comes down to some pretty straightforward math. The formulas and variables involved are about energy expenditure and work performed. These variables include frequency, intensity, time, and type.

When you make changes to one variable, you must also change another to balance the equation. Thus, if you decrease the duration (time) of each exercise session, you must increase the frequency. In another example, you could increase the intensity and decrease the duration. That's more great news.

It is truly all about working smarter, not harder. There is nothing magical about exercising continuously for one hour, or even for thirty minutes, for that matter. If you enjoy exercising for that long and are seeing results, perfect. Keep up the great work. If you've tried that formula before like so many others and struggled, however, there is hope. When it comes to sticking with an exercise program, shorter sessions make sense. You can fit them into your day in a way that works with your schedule.

When you pick quality exercises and do them correctly, at the right intensity and with consistency, then you will have all the ingredients you need to achieve excessive moderation. Are you ready to make exercise part of your lifestyle for a lifetime?

5

60 MINUTES

Did you ever stop and wonder why people consider an hour-long exercise session to be the Holy Grail of working out? Who exactly says so? Science? And why is doing over sixty minutes sometimes considered excessive, while doing less is described with apologetic terms like *only* and *just*?

"I walked just two miles today."

"I only did fifteen minutes on the elliptical this morning."

I have said the following daily for many years now, to friends, writers, and TV reporters, and now I'm saying it to you: you need to take those qualifiers out of your vocabulary when talking about exercise. Get rid of them forever. You are no longer allowed to use them.

As I have said before in this book—and as I will repeat over and over again because it's that darn important—every single minute counts when it comes to exercise. One minute of stretching. One set of push-ups. Walking up and down the stairs to your office every day instead of taking the elevator. It's not the length of your exercise session that matters; it's how consistent you are with your program every day, throughout the day.

When I first starting contributing to fitness magazines like *SELF*, *Women's Health*, *Men's Journal*, and *Men's Fitness* way back in the 1990s, I was often asked what simple tips I could give to help people work exercise into their daily lives. My response often included simples fixes like taking the stairs instead of the elevator, choosing a parking spot a bit farther away from wherever you are going, and walking whenever possible. These simple tips were often met with a "We've heard all this before, can you give us something new?" response from the editors. While I completely understood the desire of the magazines for fresh, sexy ideas (and I obliged accordingly), what I kept thinking was, *But no one's actually doing these tried-and-true, easy habits that can add up to make a big difference.*

Back when I lived in New York City, I would often take the subway to teach a group fitness class at a club or train a private client in their home gym. One day I was exiting the subway to enter Grand Central Terminal. There is a long, ascending escalator right next to an equally long staircase. It was rush hour, and people were scurrying like rats in every direction. The escalator was jam-packed, both with people riding wedged shoulder-to-shoulder and people impatiently waiting in line to step on. The stairs? They were almost completely empty. I was struck by the fact that so few people were willing to burn calories by taking the stairs instead of the escalator.

I also travel frequently for work and to compete in endurance races. I take long trips to places like China, South Africa, Brazil, and New Zealand, which can include flying times of twelve hours or more. What never ceases to amaze me is the number of people who get off these flights after having sat nearly motionless for almost half a day or more and then choose to use moving sidewalks and escalators rather than walk.

A huge part of the obesity epidemic comes down to two simple facts: we are moving less, and we are consuming more food—especially unhealthy food.

I just celebrated my fiftieth birthday, and it inspired me to think about all the ways technology has enabled our sedentary lifestyles. Here are but a few:

- You used to have to get up and walk to the television to change the channel. Now you can lie in a near-comatose state on the couch, moving only a thumb to find your favorite show. Even that tiny bit of movement will soon be a thing of the past as the remote control is replaced with voice recognition.
- Most garage doors used to be opened and closed manually. You had to physically get out of the car and push it up or pull it down.
- You had to leave the house and physically go to the store to buy most items. There was no internet, Amazon Prime, or GrubHub delivery service. Now you can have virtually everything you could possibly need delivered to your door in a ridiculously short amount of time. This is especially problematic with fast food. Have a hankering for a burger, a taco, or a couple of bacon, egg, and cheese sandwiches from your local deli? Years ago, you might have really wanted these foods but weren't willing or able to take the time and make the effort to go out and get them. Now in many parts of the country—especially urban areas—you can have any food you choose delivered to your doorstep in a matter of minutes.

I'm sure many of these activities seem trivial, and they account for only a small caloric expenditure. But when they are avoided all day long, day after day, the lack of movement adds up.

FIDGETING

Ever wonder why that friend of yours who can never seem to keep still but eats more than you do is on the skinnier side? One of the reasons could be the amount of fidgeting they do.

Burning calories while fidgeting falls under the process known as NEAT, an acronym for *non-exercise activity thermogenesis.*

NEAT is defined by the US National Institutes of Health as "all the energy expended with occupation, leisure time activity, sitting, standing, ambulation, toe-tapping, shoveling snow, playing the guitar, dancing, singing, washing, and more." Seemingly small amounts of movement like fidgeting can account for literally hundreds of extra calories burned every day.

So small amounts of moving *less* throughout the day can slowly pack on the pounds, while small amounts of moving *more* can keep them off. Once again, that should come as great news. Small, positive changes done repeatedly over time can lead to big results.

I want you to get rid of the erroneous belief that for a workout to matter, it has to take an hour. Or even close to an hour. We were made to move, and movement is quickly disappearing from our lives—especially for those not living in walking cities—so it is essential that we move whenever we can.

The science is simple and clear: you can break up your workouts and still reap the same reward. Once again, three ten-minute bouts of exercise have the same relative benefits as one continuous thirty-minute session.

An enormous part of the problem with people failing to engage in exercise are the mixed, confusing, and oft-changing guidelines put forth by different health organizations. Here are the current recommendations for those aged eighteen to sixty-four years old, according to the US Department of Health and Human Services (HHS) as of 2018:

> All adults should move more and sit less throughout the day. Some physical activity is better than none. Adults who sit less

> and do any amount of moderate-to-vigorous physical activity gain some health benefits.
>
> For substantial health benefits, adults should do at least 150 minutes (2 hours and 30 minutes) to 300 minutes (5 hours) a week of moderate-intensity, or 75 minutes (1 hour and 15 minutes) to 150 minutes (2 hours and 30 minutes) a week of vigorous-intensity aerobic physical activity, or an equivalent combination of moderate- and vigorous-intensity aerobic activity. Preferably, aerobic activity should be spread throughout the week. . . . Adults should also do muscle-strengthening activities of moderate or greater intensity and that involve all major muscle groups on 2 or more days a week, as these activities provide additional health benefits.

While I appreciate what the HHS is trying to say here, it's still awkwardly worded and confusing. First off, add *some* to the list of words you are forbidden to say as they relate to your exercise program. Couldn't the HSS simply replace the word *some* with a much more positive term, like *all*?

All physical activity is better than none.

Much better.

Some still sounds like it's not enough. It's less than motivational. It's also used twice in the recommendation, which is another problem:

" . . . *adults who participate in any amount of physical activity gain some health benefits.*"

Just *some*? Isn't that a good thing? In this case I would recommend taking the word out entirely.

" . . . *adults who participate in any amount of physical activity gain health benefits.*"

Am I splitting hairs here? Not a chance. If there's anything I have learned over the past thirty years in the fitness business, it's that messaging is everything. The message matters. It's not just what you say, but how you say it. It's all about motivation. There are no small steps forward when it comes to achieving your fitness goals, just steps.

In the next paragraph, when the HSS talks about substantial health benefits, the language used once again only serves to diminish the value and importance of shorter workouts. Finally, using terms like *moderate-intensity* and *vigorous-intensity* only confuses the issue even more. What exactly is a *moderate* or a *vigorous* workout?

Finally, the HHS does say toward the end of the report that there is "evolving evidence [that] research continues to support the conclusion that physical activity accumulated in bouts of at least 10 minutes can improve a variety of health-related outcomes."

All exercise matters. All movement counts. Minutes matter—not just hours.

Enough is enough. All exercise matters. All movement counts. Minutes matter—not just hours. A 2015 study published in the *American Journal of Clinical Nutrition* showed that even small increases in activity in inactive individuals can provide health benefits. The number one reason why people don't exercise is lack of time, time that you believe has to be long to be meaningful, effective, and worthwhile. If you believe that any workout that takes less than an hour to complete is not worth it, and that therefore it's just better to not work out at all, then you're throwing the proverbial baby out with the bathwater.

The great news is that you now know this is not true. The bad news is also that you know it's not true. You can no longer use the number one reason for not exercising—a lack of time—as the reason why you aren't working out. My sincere apologies . . .

6

THE POWER OF THE INTERVAL

Frequency, intensity, time, and type. These are the primary elements that you can manipulate to change your workout routine—how long, how hard, how often, and what kind of exercise you choose. In this chapter, I will discuss one way you can manipulate the intensity of your cardio workouts to maximize your time and your results: interval training.

interval: noun

1. An intervening time.
2. A pause or break in activity.

Although it may seem like something new thanks to all the recent coverage in the media, interval training has been around for decades. Professional athletes, in particular, have used interval training to improve their performance in a wide variety of sports. Interval training is an extremely efficient and effective form of cardiovascular exercise, one that confers numerous benefits.

These benefits aren't just for the elite athlete, either. Interval training is slowly being embraced by exercisers of all abilities and with varied fitness goals. Whether you are trying to lose weight, run faster, or live longer, interval training is for you.

WHAT IS IT?

Although there are now many different definitions of interval training as it applies to exercise—both cardiovascular and strength—interval training is, at its simplest form, the alternating of high efforts and low efforts. You can perform interval training with numerous forms of cardiovascular exercise, including running, cycling, swimming, rowing, and more. By alternating between these high and low efforts, you are able to accrue time at the higher intensities that would otherwise be difficult to achieve in one continuous effort.

For example, a competitive runner might do the following interval-type workout on a standard 400-meter track: a two-mile (3.2 km) easy warm-up jog, then 8 × 400s on one-lap recovery, finishing with a one-mile (1.6 km) cooldown. This means that, after the warm-up, the runner would sprint one lap and then walk one lap to recover, repeating this progression eight times. They would then jog one mile easy to recover.

Since four laps equal one mile on a standard 400-meter track, with this workout, the runner will sprint a total distance of two miles at a high intensity—an intensity that would be higher than if they tried to run two miles continuously.

There are numerous ways to perform interval training. You can do it by distance and by time. You can manipulate the ratio of work to recovery based on your fitness level and your goals. The general rule of thumb is: the shorter the interval, the higher the intensity.

According to a 2019 study by the *British Journal of Sports Medicine*, both interval training and continuous exercise of moderate intensity reduced body fat. Interval training, however, provided 28.5 percent greater reductions in total absolute fat mass.

HIIT

HIIT is an acronym for *high-intensity interval training*. Once again, this refers to the cycling of hard cardiovascular efforts with easy efforts. One common mistake people make when performing HIIT workouts is that their hard efforts are not hard enough and their easy efforts aren't easy enough. Remember my earlier discussion about exercise always being either too hard or too easy? Well, HIIT is one of the few times your goal is to actually be on the ends of that pendulum. You go hard for a short amount of time, then recover for a slightly longer amount of time.

A 2013 article published by the American College of Sports Medicine in their *ACSM's Health & Fitness Journal* concluded that high-intensity circuit training is an extremely efficient way to decrease body fat and improve insulin sensitivity, VO2max, and overall muscular fitness, using just your body weight.

The Gray Zone

While there is indeed benefit from all cardiovascular exercise, you can maximize your time and efforts by mixing up the intensities. One reason you might hit the dreaded plateau of seeing fewer results from your cardio workouts is because you spend almost all your time in this gray zone (see page 43).

The human body is an extremely smart machine and adapts rather quickly to the stresses imposed upon it. So one reason you burn fewer calories over time while doing the same type of work at the same intensity is that your body has become more efficient at that form of exercise. The better you are at performing a specific movement pattern, the less energy your body needs to get through the workout.

Tabata

One reason HIIT is all the rage right now is thanks to the popularity of tabata training. A form of HIIT, tabata is an exercise protocol named after Japanese scientist Dr. Izumi Tabata from the National Institute of Fitness and Sport in Tokyo, though he gives credit to Olympic speed skating coach Irisawa Koichi. Dr. Tabata originally conducted a study with Japanese speed skaters as his subjects, performing interval training on stationary bikes. The paper "Effects of Moderate-Intensity Endurance and High-Intensity Intermittent Training on Anaerobic Capacity and VO_2max," which Tabata authored alongside six other contributors, was published in the journal *Medicine and Science in Sports and Exercise* back in 1996.

The study involved two groups of subjects, one exercising at a moderate level of intensity for an hour and the other performing high-intensity interval training for just four minutes. The specific protocol for the HIIT group was both simple and brutal at the same time: twenty seconds done at an all-out, lung-searing effort followed by ten seconds of rest, repeated eight times through. Once again, just four minutes total workout time.

The results? Both groups made similar gains in aerobic fitness. Members of the HIIT group, however, also increased their anaerobic capacity by a whopping 28 percent.

One hour versus four minutes, with those who performed the shorter workout achieving greater benefits. Amazing. Getting more from doing less.

A caveat: the Tabata Protocol involved the subjects performing the twenty seconds of exercise at 170 percent of their VO_2max. (VO_2max is defined as the maximum amount of oxygen the body can utilize during a specified period of usually intense exercise.) What exactly does that mean? It means that they were pushing themselves really, really hard. The other group was working at 70 percent of their VO_2max, which is exponentially easier.

The great news is that you don't have to work at that super-high intensity to reap the benefits of HIIT. Once again, the goal is for you to alternate between periods of hard effort and intervals of active rest, staying out of the aforementioned gray zone. Go hard, go easy, go home.

Benefits of HIIT

Three of the top benefits of high-intensity interval training are:

1. **Time:** Significant results in a shorter amount of time. It's that simple. Working out smarter, rather than longer. When you have limited time to exercise, interval training is the answer.
2. **EPOC:** Yet another acronym, this one stands for *excess post-exercise oxygen consumption*. Also known as oxygen debt, it's one of the effects of engaging in interval workouts. According to recent research, not only do you burn a significant amount of calories during a HIIT workout itself; you also continue burning calories after your session is over as your body tries to return to homeostasis or a state of rest. Exactly how long your body is in this state and the number of calories burned are still open for debate, but the fact that you are burning any calories post-exercise is still a great thing.
3. **Belly Fat:** Research has also indicated that HIIT workouts may burn a little more abdominal fat than traditional steady-state cardio. Although the number of studies and relative percentage of belly fat burned are both on the low side, it is still a promising potential benefit.

This begs the obvious question: if interval training is so darn effective, why not do it all the time? Fantastic question. I'm glad you asked. When done correctly at the appropriate intensities, interval training is hard. It significantly taxes both your cardiovascular and your muscular systems. Even professional athletes like marathon runners generally go to the track for a hard interval workout just once per week. A good rule of thumb is that you want to follow every hard interval workout with at least one, if not two, easier cardio sessions. There is still great value to performing LISS workouts, an acronym for *low-intensity steady state*. Optimal health comes from performing a wide variety of cardiovascular and strength workouts, not just one type of workout, as many articles would lead you to believe.

HIIT works because it is challenging, which, in the world of exercise, means that it often comes with an increased chance of injury. You need to start slowly, build up gradually, and incorporate it judiciously into your overall plan.

HIIT works because it is challenging, which, in the world of exercise, means that it often comes with an increased chance of injury. You need to start slowly, build up gradually, and incorporate it judiciously into your overall plan.

The bottom line is that interval training is yet another powerful weapon in your exercise arsenal, especially when your time is limited. It is a great way to mix up your routine and keep your body challenged and your mind interested. Variation is a crucial component of a successful long-term exercise plan—so much so that it's the topic of the next chapter.

7

MIXING IT UP

If the definition of insanity is doing the same thing over and over again while expecting different results, then why do people make that very mistake when it comes to exercise? If you belong to a gym, take a good look around next time you are there. How many of the members do the exact same workout every single time they are there and look exactly the same as a result?

As I said in the previous chapter, your body adapts quickly to the stressors imposed upon it. This goes for both strength and cardio workouts alike. It goes all the way back to human evolution and Darwin's survival of the fittest. You either adapted physically to your environment, or you perished. End of story.

When you pick up heavy things repeatedly, as in strength training, your muscular system responds in a number of ways, both morphologically and neurologically. In other words, the shape and structure of your muscles will change along with your nervous system's ability to recruit those muscle fibers, both of which will make you stronger.

As far as cardio workouts are concerned, people often seem to forget that your heart is a muscle as well and is arguably the most important muscle in your body, which is why I will discuss it in greater detail in the next chapter, titled, appropriately, "The Most Important Muscle." Thus, when you do cardio workouts, you are stressing your heart muscle, which adapts accordingly by getting bigger and more efficient. As your heart becomes stronger and you become more proficient at performing your chosen form of cardiovascular exercise, you will need to vary the cardio routine periodically.

Once your body has adapted to the workout and gains have been made, if you fail to add variation to your routine, these changes will slow down and eventually stop altogether.

Once your body has adapted to the workout and gains have been made, if you fail to add variation to your routine, these changes will slow down and eventually stop altogether. Your exercise routine is no longer new and different as far as your body is concerned, so the body will have made the necessary adjustments. There is no reason to make any significant further changes. If you have been doing the same workout for an extended period of time and are not seeing the results you want, this could be the reason.

As you may have learned by now, I am all about great news. The great news is that when it comes to avoiding the dreaded plateau, the solution is not complex. It doesn't require expensive equipment or really hard workouts, either. In fact, it can be summarized in three short words: *Mix. It. Up.*

Seem too good to be true? It's not. It's sound exercise science.

If variation is not currently part of your exercise plan, it may be for one or more of the following reasons:

1. You don't realize the importance of variation.
2. You like what you are doing.
3. You have seen some results.
4. You don't know what to do.

Hopefully you are starting to realize why variation is so important to your exercise program. Working with a personal trainer can be so valuable because they provide this much-needed variation. Remember when I talked earlier about how we tend to do only one form of exercise, the one we enjoy the most and are genetically predisposed to do? Personal trainers often force you to step outside your comfort zone, putting you through workout routines that you wouldn't choose to do on your own.

You are paying them for variation.

They also hopefully possess knowledge about how to safely and effectively vary your routine. It matters not how different the workout is from what you would normally do. If they put you through that same workout over and over, your results will diminish over time.

You don't need to pay a personal trainer to add variation to your routine. All you need to really shake up your routine is to learn another acronym—yes, one more—whose components I have referenced a few times already: FITT.

- **Frequency:** How *often* you work out
- **Intensity:** How *hard* you work out
- **Time:** How *long* you work out
- **Type:** The *type* of workout itself

FREQUENCY: Frequency is the same as consistency. It is crucial to long-term success, and it's one component that people have the most difficulty achieving. When you realize your workouts don't have to be long to be effective and that frequency takes precedence over time, the narrative changes completely. It is exponentially easier to fit shorter workouts into your day, throughout the day, than it is to commit to ninety minutes or more of a gym workout, including travel time.

INTENSITY: Now that you've learned about intensity and how it should be varied, you can manipulate it based on two factors: how much time you have and your mood. When you are stressed out, there is nothing quite like a quick, hard HIIT workout to burn off negative energy and get those feel-good hormones flowing through your body.

TIME: One minute, five minutes, or one hour—all three time spans have value. The longer session is not necessarily better than the shorter. Rather, what matters most is that you make workouts of different lengths a part of your daily routine. Choosing not to exercise because you *only* have five minutes is no longer an option.

TYPE: Finally, when it comes to mixing it up, periodically change around the type of exercise you are doing. A quick story: there was a woman I would see at the gym who took a group fitness class every weekday at 5:00 p.m. She didn't go into the same group cycling studio or take the same yoga class every day. Instead, she would take whatever class was offered in the large group fitness studio, and it changed every night. Boot camp, boxing, mat Pilates, Zumba, you name it—she was there fifteen minutes early and ready to take it.

The result? She was in phenomenal shape.

Mix it up.

The Power of Variation

An exercise science term for the general idea I've been talking about is known as the Overload Principle. It basically means that, in order to increase your fitness, the body must be subjected to a load or resistance greater than one to which it is accustomed.

The operative word here is *accustomed.* The goal of mixing up your workouts by changing the frequency, intensity, time, and type is to keep your body from becoming accustomed.

The Mental Side

Mixing it up is not just beneficial for your body; it's also extremely important from a motivational standpoint. Let's be honest: no matter how much you love a certain form of exercise initially, if you only do that one type exclusively, there's a good chance that you will lose interest and enjoyment over time. Add in decreased results due to a lack of variation, and now you've got real problems. If you mix in different forms of exercise, you can prevent this almost inevitable mental (and physical) burnout while still enjoying fitness for many years to come.

Cross-Training

Cross-training is simply another way of adding variation to your fitness program by engaging in forms of exercise that also provide balance. The more types of exercise you choose, the better. Even though I have completed twenty-six Ironman triathlons to date along with more than seventy marathons and ultramarathons, one reason I am injury-free is the forced cross-training that triathlons require. Swimming, biking, and running are three forms of exercise that complement one another perfectly. Add in a little strength training and some flexibility work, and now you are hitting four of the five components of fitness.

Change the Order

Finally, when I meet someone who has been doing the same strength training program for months or years on end (sometimes even decades), I encourage them to make this one simple change to experience the power and effect of variation: change around the order of their exercises. That's it.

Without fail, they are shocked and amazed by how sore they are after making this seemingly inconsequential modification. They have done nothing new; they are still doing all of the exact same exercises, just in a different order. This pre-fatiguing of your muscles in a different manner is in itself a significant stimulus, especially when your muscles have been *accustomed* to this same routine for so long.

Unfortunately, the current trend in fitness content is to disparage other types of exercise while professing how one is the panacea for all your workout woes. "Use free weights, not machines. . . ." "Do HIIT, not steady-state cardio. . . ." "Lift light weights, not heavy ones. . . ." "Use heavy weights, not light ones. . . ."

My advice? Do them all.

8

THE MOST IMPORTANT MUSCLE

Let's face it. Most people exercise for two main reasons: vanity, and their relationship with gravity. Or, in other words, they want to look better and weigh less. Both are perfectly acceptable goals. I get it.

There is only one problem: you can look great and still be unhealthy.

We live in a society where image is everything, and never more so than now, thanks to the introduction and popularity of social media. If you look good in a bathing suit and have enough followers on Instagram, you too can be an instant "fitness expert." It doesn't matter if you can do one good push-up, run one mile comfortably, or hold a plank with perfect form for a minute. All that matters is how you look.

Remember back in chapter 3 when I discussed the five components of fitness? These unfit people generally possess only one of the five: body composition. Some of them worked to achieve their low body-fat percentage, while many others were simply blessed with the right parents and genetics. Yet again, just because they look good on the outside doesn't mean they possess any of the other four crucial components, especially cardiovascular fitness.

Heart disease remains the number one cause of death in the United States, accounting for more than six hundred thousand deaths per year and 23 percent of total deaths. This is why the following headlines drive me absolutely crazy. (And, yes, they are all actual headlines I pulled from online articles.)

"Why Cardio Is Such a Waste of Time"
"Should You Even Bother with Cardio?"
"3 Reasons Cardio Is a Waste of Time"
"Is Cardio Actually Necessary? (5 Reasons Why I Don't Do Cardio)"

Just typing these headlines raises my blood pressure. I've been in this industry far too long not to know two of the main underlying arguments behind these articles, as flawed and myopic as they may be.

1. You do hours of cardio, yet you still aren't losing weight.
2. Weight loss is all about diet, not cardio.

First of all, both of these arguments have to do solely with weight loss. For argument's sake let's accept the false premise that cardio isn't an important part of weight loss. (It is, but more on that in a moment.) So what? You should just stop doing cardiovascular exercise because the number on your scale isn't going down? Really?

One article actually opened by stating that cardio wasn't "necessary for heart health, for fat loss or for toning."

Wow. This is not only untrue, it's downright dangerous.

Once again, your heart is a muscle, one that can be and needs to be strengthened. Losing weight does not make your heart stronger or your cardiovascular system more efficient in the way that cardiovascular exercise does. Yes, you should strive to achieve a healthy body composition, one of the important five components of fitness. Being overweight has numerous negative health consequences. To ever use the term "waste of time" with cardiovascular exercise, however, is just sheer nonsense.

Since we are such visual creatures, here is a short list of the benefits of cardiovascular exercise:

1. Reduces stress
2. Improves cholesterol
3. Lowers blood pressure (with long-term cardiovascular exercise)
4. Improves sleep
5. Helps regulate blood sugar
6. Reduces certain types of chronic pain
7. Strengthens the immune system
8. Has numerous brain benefits
9. Improves mood
10. Decreases risk of numerous diseases

I want you to take a good, long look at that list. There isn't one benefit that you can see in the mirror or on a scale, is there? Not one. This list is far from complete as well.

Every single one of these benefits has strong scientific backing. This is why you can never say that cardio is a "waste of time" or "isn't working" simply because you aren't losing weight. This is one of the primary problems with the messaging about cardiovascular exercise, that the sole metric to determine its relative value is the amount of weight lost.

Even though many self-proclaimed fitness experts like to make it more complicated than it is, often because they lack any real education in exercise science, weight loss still comes down to simple science and basic math. So let me share with you a few numbers.

- To lose a pound (454 g) requires a caloric deficit of 3,500 calories (3.5 kcal).
- The average person burns roughly 100 calories while running a mile (1.6 km).
- While it obviously depends on numerous factors including the specifics of the individual and the type of cardio performed, the average person will burn roughly 400–600 calories (.4–.6 kcal) per hour while exercising.

These three facts are essential to helping you begin to understand cardiovascular exercise and weight loss.

First, most people have no idea that one pound equals 3,500 calories. Most are shocked to learn that they need to burn that many calories to lose just one pound. Yet, if you don't have this basic piece of information, it is extremely difficult to begin to understand how to design your eating and exercise program for weight loss and to realize the relative contributions of each.

Most reputable fitness professionals will recommend a weight loss goal of one to two pounds per week. Once again, when you give this recommendation to the average person, they will often argue that it's simply not enough. They want to lose more. When you then break it down, explaining how losing two pounds per week requires a caloric deficit of 1,000 calories per day, every day, their eyes grow wider. That would mean spending two hours per day running on the treadmill, seven days a week.

Let's look at it the other way: if you want to lose two pounds per week without doing any cardiovascular exercise whatsoever, then you would have to eat 1,000 fewer calories per day, every day.

Are you starting to see how the one-or-the-other option is so inherently flawed?

What if, instead of taking the exercise-only or diet-only approach, you combined the two? Using this method, to lose one pound per week, you need a caloric deficit of 500 calories per day. This can be accomplished by burning 250 calories through thirty minutes of exercise and cutting 250 calories per day, the equivalent of one soda or one large cookie. That approach doesn't require marathon workouts or a restrictive diet. It's doable, it's sensible, and it is an approach you can implement for a lifetime.

Know how many calories you burn through exercise and how many you consume in your diet. Make small adjustments in both, consistently, and you will be on your way to both weight loss and better health.

If you still don't think one pound per week is enough, then you still aren't doing the simple math. Making these relatively small changes will result in your losing fifty pounds in one year.

So when it comes to the whole cardio and weight-loss discussion, you need to understand the numbers. Know how many calories you burn through exercise and how many you consume in your diet. Make small adjustments in both, consistently, and you will be on your way to both weight loss and better health.

Finally, realize that it is exponentially easier to keep 500 calories out of your mouth than it is to burn it off through exercise. The first requires a split-second choice, whereas the second will take around an hour of continuous effort. This is the very reason why cardiovascular exercise is said to be unimportant when it comes to weight loss.

Yet as simple as the previous explanations and simple math might have been, there are two more important pieces to the cardio, healthy diet, and weight-loss puzzle.

1. BETTER FOOD CHOICES

The more you engage in cardiovascular exercise, the more likely you are to make better food choices. When you put in a good effort during your workout, the last thing you want is to undo all your hard work by grabbing a handful of cookies or a sugary drink. You start to pay more attention to calories, both the number you burn during your workouts and the amount in your snacks and meals.

This incredibly powerful behavioral shift is not talked about in the aforementioned articles denouncing the effects of cardiovascular exercise.

2. YOU FEEL BETTER

Two of the powerful benefits of cardiovascular exercise are decreasing stress while positively increasing your mood, both of which often lead to healthier eating habits. When you experience negative emotions like sadness, stress, and anger, then grabbing for sugary, processed quick fixes and overeating are common coping strategies. The more cardiovascular exercise you do, the better you will feel and the less likely it will be that you grab for the junk food. This is yet another reason why shorter workouts done frequently can be so powerful and effective.

More great news.

So enough with the misinformation and misdirection when it comes to cardiovascular exercise. You shouldn't measure its value by how much weight you lose. Realize there are literally dozens of incredible benefits other than burning calories that result from walking, swimming, riding a bike, and choosing to climb a flight of stairs rather than take the elevator. The vast majority of positive side effects can't be seen in the mirror or on your bathroom scale, but they are happening during each and every single cardio session.

When it comes to muscles it's not your biceps or your butt, your calves or your core that ultimately keep you alive. It's your heart.

Science says cardiovascular exercise can add years to your life. Now let me tell you what can add life to your years.

9

THE FOUNTAIN OF YOUTH

What if I told you I had the true secret to the fountain of youth? Something that would help put the brakes on the aging process while making you look and feel better, all at the same time? What would you pay for something that promised you all that?

Say hello to strength training.

It used to be that lifting weights was only for bodybuilders, for people whose primary goal was to gain as much muscle as possible. It conjured up mental images of people like Arnold Schwarzenegger and places like Muscle Beach in California, with overly tanned and heavily oiled men lifting enormous amounts of weight in minimal amounts of clothing.

As crazy as it sounds, it wasn't too long ago that athletes like baseball players, tennis players, and golfers avoided strength training, believing that building more muscle would negatively impact their performance.

Many women avoided the weight room like the plague, for numerous reasons. If they were in the minority who did engage in resistance training, they stuck to machines like the Nautilus circuit and wouldn't think of picking up a heavy dumbbell or barbell.

Times have certainly changed.

To say that strength training has numerous benefits would be a gross understatement. While it may seem like hyperbole to call it the fountain of youth, it is truly just that. Everyone who can—male and female, young and old, absolute beginner to elite athlete—should engage in some form of strength training program.

If the topic of strength training still makes you think of oversize bodybuilder types, then you need to rid yourself of that association immediately. If you are afraid of becoming too bulky, consider rereading my discussion of this fallacy in chapter 2. Finally, if you think strength training means having to go to the gym, working out for an hour, or lifting extremely heavy weights, think again.

As I said in the introduction to this book, the future of fitness is twofold: working out at home, and shorter workouts. Does that mean you can't go to the gym, or work out for an hour, or lift really heavy weights? Nope. You can do all that if you want. You just don't have to.

You don't have to do any of those things to reap the incredible rewards that come from strength training. Remember that my primary job as an exercise physiologist is to get you the greatest results in the shortest amount of time with the least likelihood of injury. I won't make you do any more than is necessary to get great results, nor will I subject you to movements or workouts where the risks far outweigh the rewards.

So what are the benefits of lifting weights? Here are a few of the top side effects of strength training.

INCREASED FUNCTIONAL STRENGTH: Full-body resistance workouts that increase your overall strength will make your day-to-day activities significantly easier. Carrying your baby, putting away your groceries, shoveling snow, you name it: if it involves your muscles, strength training will make all of these activities less strenuous and taxing on your body.

INCREASED ENERGY: It stands to reason that the stronger you are, the less energy you'll need for your normal activities of daily living and the more energy you will have to spare. That's what's insidious about being inactive and gaining weight. It's a horrible snowball effect. You become weaker while you get heavier, both of which make your daily tasks harder and harder.

DECREASED LIKELIHOOD OF INJURY: This benefit of strength training is so very important for living a full and vibrant life. When you have muscle weaknesses and imbalances, dysfunction is often the result. Numerous musculoskeletal issues result from these two factors, including injuries to the knees, shoulders, hips, lower back, and more. Strong muscles create essential support for your joints. The weaker the muscles are around a joint, the greater the likelihood of injury.

Just think of the number of people who slip and fall when they are older, often fracturing a bone, such as a hip, in the process. Strength training will not only decrease your likelihood of falling in the first place; it will also potentially decrease the severity of your injuries if you do.

DECREASED PAIN: So many people live with pain and discomfort each and every day, pain that can often be remedied by fixing their weak links through strength training. I should know; I have spent almost three decades doing just that with countless clients, family, and friends. Once again, common ailments like back pain and shoulder issues are often remedied through a few simple exercises.

INCREASED METABOLISM: This one should get you really excited. The more muscle you have, the higher your metabolism, and thus the more calories you burn twenty-four hours a day, seven days a week. Adding lean muscle is one of the only natural ways in which you can truly boost your metabolism naturally.

Muscle tissue is more metabolically active than fat tissue, which means that the more you have, the better when it comes to losing and maintaining your weight.

COMBATS SARCOPENIA: What the heck is sarcopenia? It's the fancy term for the gradual loss of muscle mass. The average person, regardless of gender, begins to lose muscle starting in their thirties, which is known as *sarcopenia*. If there's one thing that speeds up the aging process and decreases your quality of life, it's sarcopenia.

But there is one piece of truly great news when it comes to a specific benefit of a form of exercise: *strength training can slow down and even reverse the effects of sarcopenia.* You need to understand it, embrace it, get excited about it, and then begin to apply it.

Sarcopenia is one of the primary causes of functional decline as we age. The less muscle we have, the less our body is able to do what we ask of it. It makes such complete sense, yet so few realize how crucial it is to strength train.

A 2010 study published in the journal of *Clinical Interventions in Aging* found that pharmaceutical drugs have shown limited effectiveness in combatting sarcopenia; resistance training, on the other hand remains the most effective intervention. This review also shows that it's never too late to start and that positive changes can be made by strength training, even in the elderly and infirm.

In my experience, people fail to embrace strength training for four reasons:

1. They don't realize the benefits.
2. They don't think they have the time.
3. They don't know what to do.
4. They become injured while doing it.

Enough is enough. Now you know a few of the invaluable benefits, and I will list a few more shortly. Time is no longer an issue, because I will give you five-minute strength training workouts, many of which you can do without equipment, anytime and anywhere, and which can completely change your life. Don't know what to do? How about thirty different micro-workouts that you can follow, step-by-step, as well as combine in an almost infinite number of ways to keep you motivated and seeing results? If you have tried strength training and became injured as a result, you are far from alone. My workouts and progressive approach can not only help rehabilitate many common issues but can also minimize the chance that they will happen again.

As if all these benefits weren't enough, here are a handful more:

- **Decreased Depression:** Studies have shown that, like cardiovascular exercise, lifting weights helps to combat depression and improve mood states.
- **Control Abdominal Fat:** Yes, it's true. Research has shown that, thanks to the metabolically active properties of muscle tissue, strength training is effective for preventing increases in abdominal fat.
- **Reduced Risk of Certain Cancers:** Abdominal fat, also known as visceral fat, can increase the risk of certain types of cancer. Once again, strength training can help to control the accumulation of this dangerous visceral fat.
- **Increased Cardiovascular Health:** Lifting weights helps to increase your body's levels of good cholesterol, HDL, which has heart health benefits.
- **Improved Blood Sugar Levels:** Strength training increases the body's ability to take in and use glucose, which is why it is an important intervention for people with type 2 diabetes.

- **Healthy Body Image:** Last but not least, lifting weights helps to sculpt your body, making you look better and feel better about yourself. We are and will always be visual creatures. Wanting to improve your appearance is a perfectly acceptable reason to start lifting weights. However, you need to realize that, as is also true of cardiovascular exercise and weight loss, strength training provides many other important benefits besides those you see in the mirror.

Take a look back at the myriad benefits of strength training and truly understand how important it is to build muscle and stay strong as you age. Muscle is absolutely essential to your quality of life.

Studies published in numerous medical journals from the fields of geriatrics, sports medicine, physical fitness, and cardiology show that:

- A combination of aerobic exercise and strength training improved cognitive function, muscle endurance, aerobic conditioning, and balance in older adults with moderate cognitive impairment. Moderate- and high-intensity strength training programs had equally beneficial effects on cognitive functioning.
- Strength training in the elderly is an effective way to both prevent muscle loss and retain motor function, even when using higher intensities.
- Resistance training enhances psychological well-being in older women, significantly, and total body strength training, including high-intensity training, can help improve their balance, whether the women are healthy or in an exercise rehabilitation program.

- Both cardiovascular exercise and strength training programs have positive effects on sleep quality in middle-aged and older adults.
- Low-intensity strength training can combat the negative effects of decreased daily steps in the elderly, increasing strength and decreasing the loss of muscle mass.
- Strength training can benefit memory among older adults, especially if they use higher resistance levels, and strength training can also improve memory performance in sedentary elderly individuals with prior memory issues, in addition to increasing muscle strength.
- Strength training can be as effective as aerobic exercise in improving physical skills that contribute to functional mobility and quality of life in later years. Another finding was that strength training also had positive effects on mood.
- A study conducted by the *Journal of Cachexia, Sarcopenia and Muscle* in June 2014 was one of the first to show that strength training and the increase in muscle mass helped reduce systemic inflammation in older adults with type 2 diabetes.

Here's the absolute truth about strength training: you will either do it because you want to or because you have to. It's not a matter of if, but when. Don't believe me? It's true, and I'll explain exactly why in the next chapter.

10

PREHAB VS. REHAB

Perhaps you've been to a physical therapist and that's one reason you are reading this book. Maybe you're currently working with a therapist. Every day I speak to people who have been to physical therapy numerous times, often for the same frustrating, recurring injury.

So please allow me to say it once again: if you think you can avoid lifting weights, you're mistaken. You will either engage in strength training proactively, while you are healthy and for all the reasons I outlined in the previous chapter, or you will do it *reactively* once you have become injured and while paying a physical therapist for the privilege.

The choice is completely yours.

I call it "prehab vs. rehab." What I realized many years ago while working as a personal trainer was that the workouts prescribed for people who are injured were the very same ones they should be doing while healthy. Doing these exercise routines while healthy helps to bulletproof your body, creating strength and stability that significantly decreases your chance of injury.

Take the shoulder, for example. Chances are good that you may have experienced a shoulder injury over the years. The shoulder complex is the most mobile joint in the body, and with that freedom of movement comes instability and a much higher likelihood of injury. Injuries to the rotator cuff, a group of muscles and tendons that support the shoulder joint, are extremely common.

Sports that involve throwing, like baseball and softball, racket sports like tennis, certain Olympic barbell movements, and sports like swimming all involve repetitive overhead motions that place significant strain on the shoulder joint. Engaging in these activities with weak shoulder muscles is almost a guarantee of eventual pain, discomfort, injury, and the potential need for surgery.

The same holds true with the knee joint. I have had hundreds of people discuss their "bad knees" with me over the years when they find out I am an exercise physiologist. ACLs, MCLs, meniscus tears—I am meeting more people who need knee surgeries at younger ages than ever before.

These issues are not limited to sports, either: activities of daily living often result in injuries to the joints, both acute and chronic.

Once again it comes down to human nature: you don't appreciate that you are injury-free until you start to have problems. You blame your issues on getting older or an injury or simple bad luck. Although some injuries are indeed freak accidents and unavoidable, a huge percentage are completely within your control.

More great news.

As I discussed earlier, our bodies are becoming weaker and weaker thanks to all the advances in technology. Think about how many hours each day you spend motionless: lying in bed, driving in your car, sitting at your desk, and lying on the couch. It's truly frightening. This insane amount of inactivity is wreaking havoc on your body, decreasing your functional strength and thus making you more susceptible to injury.

Hip injuries and lower back pain are two more extremely common issues today, both of which can be significantly minimized through preventative strength training. As the saying goes, an ounce of prevention is worth a pound of cure. Strengthen your muscles now so that you don't have to rehabilitate them later.

A study published in the *Journal of Applied Physiology* in 1985 showed that lifelong strength training has a protective effect against age-related loss of neuromuscular function.

A more recent study from 2006, published in the *Arthritis & Rheumatology* journal, found that strength training increased strength while decreasing the negative progression of knee osteoarthritis in subjects whose mean age was sixty-nine.

I cannot stress strongly enough how doing a few minutes of preventative exercises consistently can make a world of difference. That is the very reason I opened the book with the story of Bill; he is a perfect example and real-world proof of how a program focused on prehab can help you be injury-free and in the best shape of your life, regardless of your prior issues, even in your later years.

Especially in your later years.

My five-minute workouts are exactly what you need to bulletproof your body. Their primary goal is to create functional strength in your entire body, from your head down to your toes. They will also help build lean muscle and improve the way you look, but my first goal is always to fix the weak links and imbalances.

Why is this so important? Because being injury-free is paramount for long-term health. As they say, life is a marathon, not a sprint. Just because you can do a really difficult workout today doesn't mean you should. In fact, the current trend is to do just that: exercises and workouts where the risks far outweigh the rewards, where the skill and strength required exceed the relative abilities of the participants. The end result? Injury.

Once again, the solution is excessive moderation. Don't do a lot of exercise a little, do a little bit a lot. Five minutes of purposeful, targeted exercises. Once you become injured, you often have to stop working out for an extended period in order to heal. If the injury is severe enough, it may prevent you from participating in the activities you enjoy, sometimes forever.

Don't do a lot of exercise a little, do a little bit a lot. Five minutes of purposeful, targeted exercises.

I have been in the fitness industry long enough to understand one thing: getting you to embrace and then implement the concept of prehab is one of my biggest challenges. It doesn't involve losing weight or sculpting your ideal physique. It's not something you can measure or quantify. It's not about achieving a number on the scale, finally being able to hold a plank for a minute, or running your first 5K.

Success comes from something *not* happening, namely avoiding pain and injury.

This is why at the beginning of this book I said that you cannot achieve true health and wellness without truly believing in the process. You have to have faith that what you are doing is worthwhile. That it matters.

It is so easy to become complacent when you are feeling good and have no major aches and pains. You need to realize that this state of being is earned, especially as you grow older. It's not guaranteed, and it's not luck.

Luck

If *bulk* is my least favorite word in the world of fitness, *luck* comes in a close second. Back when I was coaching athletes to participate in races, I would never wish them good luck before an event. They either did the work or they didn't. It wasn't about luck. It was about doing the work, putting in the time, and then executing their plan.

I recently traveled to New Zealand to celebrate turning fifty by participating in my twenty-sixth Ironman triathlon. I wrote a post on the experience and how I was most proud of having never had a major injury after twenty years of racing endurance events around the world. One person commented on the article by saying they would "knock on wood for me" to help me avoid becoming injured in the future. While I understand and appreciate the sentiment, it's not luck that has kept me from having to step foot in a physical therapist's office after all those races and after all those miles in training. It's certainly not from knocking on wood.

What has kept me healthy is prehab. Excessive moderation. Believing that the work I am doing is worthwhile, even though I don't see visible results. My primary goal is to remain injury-free so that I can continue to enjoy life to its fullest.

It goes back to my earlier discussion about control. Either you believe you have control over your health—significant control—or you don't. The main focus of this book is to illustrate that very point. Hopefully, I have been successful in my efforts.

You have to believe in the science, trust the process, be consistent, and give it time. If you do these four things, I promise you great things will happen.

Let's face it: it's a pretty big stretch to believe that after twenty-six Ironman races, more than seventy marathons and ultramarathons, and literally hundreds of other races, my injury avoidance comes down to luck. Especially since I spent the majority of my time participating in youth sports on the bench, unable to run thanks to numerous musculoskeletal issues.

You have to believe in the science, trust the process, be consistent, and give it time. If you do these four things, I promise you great things will happen. I am living proof, as are those who have followed my plans over the years.

Finally, one of the major challenges with strengthening your weak links is that the exercises can be boring. I completely understand. They generally don't involve particularly fun or exciting movements. You won't be standing with one foot on a balance disc while slamming a sandbag on the floor, jumping up and down on a plyometric box while wearing a weight vest, or seeing how many reps of an advanced exercise you can do every minute, on the minute.

If strengthening exercises were especially exciting, everyone would do them and we would have far fewer injured people as a result. Just realize that I'm not asking you to do an hour of these exercises or even a half hour. All I'm asking for is five minutes. Five minutes, done consistently, will help bulletproof your body by strengthening your weak links and correcting muscular imbalances, allowing you to enjoy life to the fullest.

11

FOCUS ON THE NEGATIVE

My first real fitness job was working in a Nautilus facility during one summer in college. It was one room within my local YMCA, complete with a full circuit of Nautilus machines lining the perimeter. I was trained on how to use each one and spent three months managing the facility and teaching people the proper way to use the equipment.

That summer was a true turning point in my life on a number of levels. Even though I had already embraced exercise years earlier, doing push-ups and working out down in my makeshift home gym, I realized how much I also enjoyed working in a gym environment. I loved everything about it: working with people of all fitness levels and abilities, teaching people what I had learned about exercise, and, yes, using the equipment myself whenever I could.

Of course, when the club was empty, I would work out myself.

I got on those machines whenever the opportunity presented itself. The circuit worked your entire body, with each machine targeting one specific major muscle group: chest, back, shoulders, triceps, biceps, hamstrings, quadriceps, and abdominals.

I absolutely transformed my body that summer.

The Nautilus protocol utilized one to three sets of eight to twelve repetitions, where the last few repetitions should be difficult without losing proper form. If you couldn't do eight repetitions, then the weight was too heavy. When the last few became easy, it was time to increase the resistance.

Last, I was taught to use a two-second/four-second repetition when performing an exercise. This meant that the concentric phase of an exercise, the raising of the weight, should be done for a two-count, while the lowering back down—the eccentric or "negative" phase—should be performed a little more slowly, taking four seconds to complete. For instance, when using the chest-press machine, you push the handles away from your body with a two count, then take four seconds to lower it back down.

As crazy as it may sound, that six-second repetition is one of the major "secrets" to success with my fitness program. I started doing it in those early college days, and I am still using that simple formula today. The major premise is that the "negative" part of resistance training is extremely important.

MOST PEOPLE ARE DOING IT BACKWARD

If you watch people lifting weights at the gym, you'll see that the vast majority do it completely backward. They swing the weights up on a rough two-count, then drop them back down quickly, letting gravity do the majority of the work, taking about a second to return to the starting position. This happens with free weights, machines, during bodyweight exercises, and more.

Take a basic push-up, for example. It is seldom that I see someone do a push-up with correct form. Most often they are more pulses than push-ups, done too fast and with a limited range of motion.

Here's a fun little exercise for you: try doing a push-up using the two-second/four-second method. Lower yourself down to the floor while counting slowly to four; then raise yourself back up while counting to two, ending the movement with your arms fully extended.

Try it right now and see how many you can do. My guess is that you will be surprised by how challenging it is to do a basic push-up using this simple technique.

I use the six-second repetition rule for almost all my strength exercises, regardless of the modality. Machines, free weights, body weight, resistance bands, you name it. Bicep curls with dumbbells, cable rows, body-weight squats—all with the "down" a little slower than the "up." I sometimes use a two-second/three-second repetition, but the negative is always slower.

Time-Under-Tension

When you slow the repetition down in this manner, you decrease the relative contribution of momentum while increasing the muscle's time under tension. It's really difficult—almost impossible actually—to lower the weight back down on a two- to four-count without keeping the targeted muscles engaged.

More muscle engagement means more work performed, which gives you increased results. You will get more out of each exercise and more from each workout.

DOMS

Time for another acronym. DOMS stands for *delayed onset muscle soreness.* Anyone who has worked out in the past knows exactly what this is. Remember when you did your first hard leg workout and how you were a little sore the next day, but then you could barely walk the day after that? This is known as DOMS, and it usually presents forty-eight hours after a new or particularly strenuous workout. It is the result of tiny microtears in your muscle tissue that occur primarily during the eccentric or negative phase of each exercise. DOMS generally happens when first starting a challenging, brand-new exercise program, and the soreness usually subsides after about 24 hours or so.

DON'T FIXATE ON THE NUMBER OF REPETITIONS

I really don't care how much weight I can lift, and I couldn't care less how many push-ups I can do. What matters to me most when it comes to my workouts is the quality of each and every exercise, not the quantity of the repetitions or how much I can bench press. I would much rather do twenty-five slow, controlled push-ups than fifty bad ones. When I see someone cranking out endless basic crunches, I know immediately that their goal is simply to do a specific number of repetitions. How do I know this? Simply by the manner in which the exercise is done: with fast, partial repetitions using significant momentum and minimal muscle engagement.

I was asked not too long ago to take part in a push-up contest. I politely declined, not because I didn't think I had a decent chance of winning, but because I knew that I would have to do the push-ups with poor form in order to participate.

So much of strength training has to do with ego, especially when working out in a gym with others. Ask yourself this: is your goal to impress others for an hour at your club a few times a week, or is it to be functionally strong and injury-free for a lifetime?

USE MODERATELY HEAVY WEIGHTS

Slowing down your repetitions not only forces you to keep the tension on the muscle, making the exercise more challenging; it also requires the use of slightly lighter weights. Not light weights, but *lighter* weights—most likely lighter than you are used to: weights that are challenging for the last few repetitions without making you sacrifice proper form while performing this slower lifting protocol. You can use heavier weights when you swing them up and down quickly, using momentum and gravity to do a large amount of the work. If you normally do your bicep curls at a fast pace with fifty-pound dumbbells, try using the same weight while doing six-second repetitions. In order to do the same amount of repetitions, you'll probably have to swap out the fifties for a pair of forties, or possibly less. Yet the lighter weight doesn't mean you are getting less out of the exercise; you are actually getting more.

Greater Results with Less Likelihood of Injury

Remember when I said (several times) that my primary job is to get you the greatest results in the shortest amount of time? Well, when it comes to strength training, that means focusing on the negative. Using weights that are too heavy significantly increases your risk of injury. Using momentum increases your risk of injury. Using poor form—you get the picture.

So use moderately heavy weights, slow down each repetition, and keep constant tension on the muscles you are trying to target. This will decrease your likelihood of injury while increasing your results. Say it with me now: more great news.

Use moderately heavy weights, slow down each repetition, and keep constant tension on the muscles you are trying to target.

Even though I spend my life looking on the positive side of things, when it comes to strength training, I focus on the negative.

Can I tell you the greatest compliment I receive while lifting weights at the gym, one that I get all the time? What do you think it might be? I guarantee you haven't the slightest chance of getting it right. None.

It's actually a question, usually just three words: "Are you hurt?"

Now I'm sure you think I am completely nuts. How can this possibly be a positive thing, much less a compliment?

It can, because it shows that I am actually practicing exactly what I preach. First and foremost, those who ask if I am hurt do so because I have a significant amount of lean muscle, yet I use lighter weights. They cannot believe that I have achieved my physique without lifting much heavier weights. It can't be possible.

Second, they see me doing my prehab exercises, like internal and external shoulder rotation. Many have done these exercises themselves in physical therapy, so they immediately assume I am coming back from an injury myself.

Try slowing down your repetitions during your next strength workout. See how different and more challenging a six-second repetition feels. Use lighter weights, focus on the quality of each movement, and give it time. You will be amazed by the results.

A final fun fact: twenty-five years after starting my very first fitness job in that Nautilus facility, I was hired by Nautilus, Inc. to be a Bowflex Fitness Advisor. Talk about coming full circle.

12

JOHN'S STORY

I started working with John back in 2005, when he was in his early fifties. I was still working as a personal trainer at the time, doing private sessions at people's homes in Connecticut. John's wife hired me as a birthday present for him.

Like most men in their late forties and early fifties, John had spent the past few decades focused on his work and not his health. He was an entrepreneur who had built an extremely successful business from the ground up, which required long hours and a significant amount of international travel.

Now his body was beginning to break down. He was overweight, his triglycerides were elevated, and he was taking medication to treat his cholesterol. He lacked energy, and his flexibility was horrible. There was much work to be done.

John wasn't doing any strength training whatsoever. He didn't belong to a gym and didn't own one piece of home exercise equipment. However, he had recently started walking a few times per week, a few miles at a time, thanks to his wife's encouragement.

John could barely do a few push-ups, and a basic bodyweight squat posed a significant challenge. His hamstrings and lower back were ridiculously tight, and he couldn't come close to touching his toes as a result. I explained to him how it was going to take a significant amount of time to achieve his goals, how he had to trust the process, and how he had to be consistent with our workouts. John agreed with all I asked of him, and I could tell he was extremely motivated and focused on achieving his goals.

We decided that we would work out together four times per week at his home, doing a combination of strength work and cardiovascular exercise. We started slowly, as you would expect. We didn't use any equipment for many weeks and just focused on basic bodyweight exercises and building a base of strength. We progressed to light dumbbells and then to resistance bands, keeping it simple.

One of John's goals was to be able to run a few miles continuously, something that he had never been able to do before, so for our cardio sessions we went outside and began to work on his cardiovascular endurance. When we went out for our very first workout, John could run for only 30 to 60 seconds at a time, so we began with the run/walk method I had used with hundreds of other clients. We would run slowly for thirty seconds or so, then walk for three to five minutes to recover. We would repeat this progression for the duration of the cardio session, which was roughly twenty minutes to start.

To say it wasn't easy for John would be a gross understatement. Years of sitting at a desk all day long and on planes for hours on end had significantly weakened his cardiovascular system. It had also taken a toll on his leg muscles; John began to experience all the common aches and pains associated with running.

He never gave up, however. He believed in himself and his ability to achieve every goal we had written down for him during our initial consultation. When he would start to feel discomfort, I would determine the cause and we would deal with it immediately, before it became an issue or an injury. John never used these inevitable temporary obstacles as a reason to give up.

As John improved his cardiovascular fitness, I would gradually increase his run interval while decreasing the amount of time he walked. Very gradually. I would also slowly lengthen our cardio sessions as his endurance improved.

We stretched. We strengthened. We did a little of everything rather than a lot of any one thing. We wor ked on all five of the components of fitness, implementing all the principles I have outlined up until this point.

John not only eventually achieved all his goals; he blew them completely out of the water.

We worked on all five of the components of fitness, implementing all the principles I have outlined up until this point.

John not only eventually achieved all his goals; he blew them completely out of the water.

Once he was able to run thirty minutes without stopping, I convinced him to sign up for his first 5K race. It wasn't easy, but he finished. We continued to build his strength, discovering and correcting his muscular imbalances and weaknesses.

That first 5K led to more 5Ks. Then 10Ks. What was astonishing was that, as John began to bulletproof his body and build balanced, total body strength, we learned that not only could he run longer and longer distances, but he was actually fast.

Really fast.

Three years after we shuffled through our very first thirty-second "run," John and I ran the Paris Marathon together. He was fifty-six years old and finished in a more-than-respectable four hours and twenty-five minutes. Incredible. His daughter ran it with us too.

John continued to run races of all distances, including more marathons. He became incredibly focused on getting stronger, faster, and fitter. Incredibly, he qualified for the Boston Marathon and then, five years after running his very first marathon and at age sixty-one, John set a personal record for himself. He ran the Boston Marathon again, this time in three hours and forty-three minutes. That's an average of an eight-and-a-half-minute mile for twenty-six miles.

Beyond incredible. The man who could barely run a minute, much less a mile, at age fifty had suddenly become a competitive age-group distance runner at age sixty.

But his story doesn't end there.

John also embraced the concept of variation. As healthy as running was for him, I encouraged him to mix things up. He soon added cycling to his routine, beginning with short rides around town. As with his running, he progressed slowly. His wife also bought a bike, and the two began to go out for short rides after work and longer rides on the weekend.

A few years after John added cycling as part of his cross-training routine, he biked across the entire country, from Los Angeles to Boston—3,450 miles (5,550 km) in total. His wife even joined him for a significant portion of the ride.

Fast-forward to today. John's athletic resume includes thirteen marathons, more than three dozen half marathons, and countless 5Ks and 10Ks. In addition to the cross-country ride, he has also biked the following:

- London to Rome (2,000 miles [3,218 km])
- Canada to Mexico (1,200 miles [1,930 km])
- Venice to Salzburg (1,000 miles [1,610 km])

Today, John is still going strong. This summer he'll bike 2,000 miles, from Barcelona to Rome.

I still have the initial questionnaire I had John fill out during our first meeting. Under the heading "Fitness Goals," he listed the following:

1. Lose 20 pounds (9 kg)
2. Lower triglycerides
3. Increase flexibility

He achieved all three and a whole heck of a lot more.

John was and still is one of my most incredible success stories as a trainer and coach. Like Bill in chapter 1, John embraced all of the principles I have outlined in these pages. He put in the work, he gave it time, and he is living his best life. He is healthy enough to enjoy life to the fullest, traveling and exploring the world by foot and by bike.

John is not an outlier. He didn't get lucky. He did the work, and he will be reaping the rewards for many years to come.

So can you.

13
SUSAN STRONG

I met Susan in the conference room of her family business to conduct our initial consultation. An extremely busy executive in her late forties, Susan had been working tirelessly for years and was now positioned to take over the decades-old, multimillion-dollar company. We spent the better part of two hours discussing her current fitness plan, injury history, goals, current schedule, and more. Not only did Susan's job come with a six-day work-week, long hours, and a high level of stress, but she was also the mother of three young children.

Susan admitted that she smoked, she didn't exercise regularly, and her eating habits left much room for improvement. Yet, like the vast majority of the top executives I have worked with over the years, Susan knew that she was at a pivotal turning point in her life. She needed to improve her lifestyle if she wanted to continue to not only maintain her current chaotic schedule but also take her success to the next level.

Her goals were like those of most people: she wanted to lose some weight, tighten and tone several problem areas, and fix a few nagging injuries. These weren't her focus, however. Susan's primary goal, the main reason she was hiring me to work with her, was to increase her energy and mental focus. She knew that regular exercise was essential to her not only being able to handle the physical demands of her job, but the mental requirements as well. Susan also realized that working out would help her better cope with the added stressors of being a busy working mother.

Susan was not one to do something halfway, which was one of the reasons she had already achieved a high level of success. Whereas most people who work with a trainer do so once or twice a week, three times a week at most, Susan wanted to train five days a week. At five in the morning.

Although she was not a runner, Susan knew that I made running part of the training with certain clients and expressed interest in doing it herself. Like John, however, Susan stated that she could run for only a short time before becoming winded and having to walk. I put together a program that included a combination of short runs outside along with bodyweight and dumbbell exercises at home.

We started slowly: some days we would focus on walk/run workouts, while others entailed foundational strength work at her home. Often the hour would include a combination of the two. We started with the basics and progressed slowly, using the very same exercises found in the thirty micro workout section of this book (see pages 97–100).

Susan possessed one trait that was shared by every single one of my clients who achieved (and often exceeded) their initial fitness goals—she showed up. Cancellations were extremely rare, and if a session was canceled, it was rescheduled rather than missed completely. Susan, Bill, and John all realized how incredibly important consistency was for achieving their goals.

Susan possessed one trait that was shared by every single one of my clients who achieved (and often exceeded) their initial fitness goals—she showed up.

They may not have called it that, but they were all practicing excessive moderation.

Not only did Susan and I run outdoors at five in the morning, we did it all year long, even in the dead of winter, regardless of the conditions. I vividly remember looking at the temperature reading on my car dashboard and seeing 9 degrees as I pulled up in the pitch dark to begin yet another chilly workout.

Pouring rain? We ran. Ninety-eight degrees and humid? We ran. Late night out? We ran. No excuses.

Slowly but surely the strength and cardio workouts began to pay off. Susan began to lose weight. She added muscle and improved her strength. She cut her smoking down considerably, indulging only a few times a month. Those nagging aches and pains were all but forgotten. Susan began making better food choices, and her energy levels improved considerably.

After a few months of consistent work, Susan had significantly increased her running endurance. We would run a mile and then walk for sixty seconds, repeating this pattern for several miles. At the end of one of our frigid morning runs I suggested we run a 5K together, and she agreed immediately.

For someone who had described herself as "not a runner" during our initial meeting, Susan successfully completed her first 5K after just a few months of training and with a huge smile on her face. Forever the goal-setter and someone who now realized how these events gave her workouts purpose, Susan suggested we train for a 10K.

As you might expect, a few months later we crossed the finish line of that 10K race. Susan had lost even more weight since the 5K and had added more lean muscle. She was feeling strong and empowered.

Here's where Susan's story takes a little turn.

After the race, her husband walked up to us and I said to him, "You know, I think Susan could run a marathon."

He laughed for a few seconds and then replied, "She'll never run a marathon." Not the right thing to say to a woman with Susan's drive.

Within the next few years, Susan completed not one, but five marathons. We ran the New York City Marathon, the Chicago Marathon, and the Rock 'n' Roll Marathon in San Diego. We shuffled through the Boston Marathon in sweltering 86-degree heat.

For her final marathon, we flew to Italy and ran the Rome Marathon, starting and finishing at the Colosseum.

Susan no longer runs marathons, and she's no longer married to the man who questioned her abilities. She is focused on running the family business as the new CEO, following the excessive moderation guidelines for her exercise plan, and getting in frequent shorter workouts in the new home gym we designed for her. She's stronger, she's healthier, and she's happier, having far exceeded the goals we had originally set for her.

14

THIRTY 5-MINUTE MICRO WORKOUTS

Enough talk about the *why*, now let's talk about the *what*. What workouts are you going to do to get rid of those nagging aches and pains, fix your weak links, and strengthen you from head to toe, adding years to your life and life to your years?

Thirty different 5-minute workouts.

There are ten categories of workouts, each with three progressively challenging versions. If you are just starting out, begin with the first workout in each category. Once you feel comfortable with the movements and have built up your strength, move on to the second workout in the category, then the third.

You will never outgrow a workout, however. I still do all thirty of these myself.

You can add additional resistance, like dumbbells, to the bodyweight exercises (squats, stationary lunges, step-ups, etc.) if you need a greater challenge. Just be sure not to do so too soon, and make sure you are still performing the exercise with good form and through a full range of motion.

Stacking Workouts

You can do each 5-minute workout on its own, throughout your day. For example, you can do a 5-minute cardio workout in the morning before you get in the shower, a 5-minute ab workout in your office in the afternoon, and then a 5-minute total body workout before the kids get home from school.

You can also "stack" several of the workouts back-to-back if you'd like, whenever you have more time. They are designed to be combined in an almost infinite number of ways based on your goals, how much time you have available, and what you feel like doing that day.

The exercises are done by time, not by number of repetitions. They vary from 15 to 75 seconds each. The goal is not to do as many repetitions as possible but to go slowly and do what you are capable of with good form. Generally speaking, however, try to use a 3- to 4-second repetition (1 second for the "up," 2 to 3 seconds for the "down") when the exercise calls for 30 seconds, which should result in about 10 repetitions. Try to go a little slower for the 60-second exercises, using the 2-second/4-second repetition methodology. (Note: The 15-second exercise intervals are for stretches and the 75 for cardio intervals, so no repetitions are involved.)

Finally, you do have the option of doing any of the same workouts several more times through if you so choose; you could make a workout 7.5 minutes (3 rounds) or 10 minutes (4 rounds of 2.5 minutes).

The workouts are categorized as follows:

- 5-Minute Cardio
- 5-Minute Core
- 5-Minute Abs
- 5-Minute Upper Body
- 5-Minute Lower Body
- 5-Minute Arms
- 5-Minute Lower Back
- 5-Minute Total Body
- 5-Minute Rx
- 5-Minute Stretch

The 30 workouts are divided into three progressively more difficult phases. Beginners should start with Phase 1, performing it until they feel comfortable with all the movements before progressing to Phase 2 and likewise to Phase 3.

That being said, even intermediate to advanced exercisers will benefit from performing all of the exercises, including those found in Phase 1. Variation of all three phases will allow you to maintain your fitness, add the variety needed to keep your body from plateauing, and help to avoid boredom and burnout from performing the same workouts over and over.

30 MICRO WORKOUTS

PHASE 1	PHASE 2	PHASE 3
Cardio 1	Cardio 2	Cardio 3
Core 1	Core 2	Core 3
Abs 1	Abs 2	Abs 3
Upper Body 1	Upper Body 2	Upper Body 3
Lower Body 1	Lower Body 2	Lower Body 3
Arms 1	Arms 2	Arms 3
Lower Back 1	Lower Back 2	Lower Back 3
Total Body 1	Total Body 2	Total Body 3
Rx Shoulders	Rx Knees	Rx Lower Back
Stretch 1	Stretch 2	Stretch 3

Here are a few examples of how you might structure a week of workouts. Once again, these workouts can be done back-to-back or separately throughout the day.

SAMPLE WEEK 1

MO	TU	WE	TH	FR	SA	SU
Cardio	Core	Upper Body	Cardio	Total Body	Cardio	Stretch
Total Body	Rx Shoulders	Lower Body	Abs	Stretch	Rx Knees	
Abs						

SAMPLE WEEK 2

MO	TU	WE	TH	FR	SAT	SU
Core	Cardio	Rx Shoulders	Total Body	Stretch	Total Body	Rx Shoulders
Upper Body	Lower Body	Rx Knees	Cardio		Cardio	Rx Knees
Stretch		Rx Back	Stretch			Rx Back

SAMPLE WEEK 3

MO	TU	WE	TH	FR	SA	SU
Upper Body	Core	Total Body	Core	Total Body	Cardio	Rx Back
Lower Body	Cardio	Core	Cardio	Stretch		Lower Back
Abs		Abs		Abs		
		Stretch		Cardio		

As you can see, there are a wide variety of ways you can mix and match these workouts. Have fun with them and mix them up.

Believe in yourself, be consistent, and remember—five minutes matters.

15

5-MINUTE EXERCISE ROUTINES

So here you have it: thirty different 5-minute workouts. Each set of exercises is 2.5 minutes in length, so perform two rounds of each for a five-minute workout. If you need a few seconds' rest in between exercises or rounds, take it.

The stretches are either 2.5 or 5 minutes in length. Do the 2.5-minute stretches two times through to equal a full five minutes.

You can mix and match them any way you choose, based on your available time, the body parts you wish to work, your fitness level, and the way you decide to structure your week. Always remember that the goal in excessive moderation is doing something every day (with one day of rest if you'd like.)

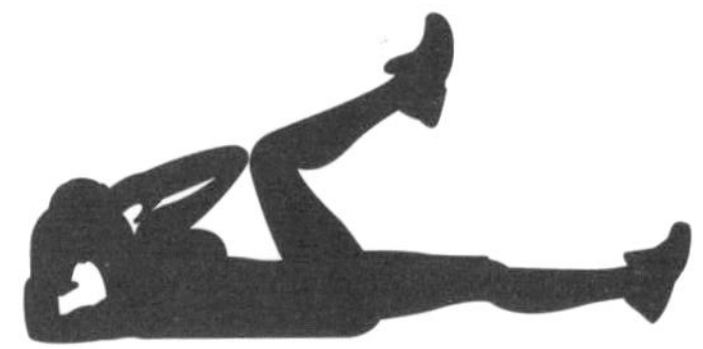

5-MINUTE AB WORKOUTS

ABS 1

- Hand Crunches (30 seconds)
- Bent Knee Oblique Crunch (30 seconds each side)
- Straight Arm Plank (30 seconds)
- Jabs (30 seconds)

ABS 2

- Regular Crunch (30 seconds)
- Side Oblique Crunch (30 seconds each side)
- Reverse Crunch (30 seconds)
- Bicycle Crunch (30 seconds)

ABS 3

- Cross-Crunch (30 seconds)
- Double Crunch (30 seconds)
- Side Scissors Crunch (30 seconds each side)
- Tuck Jumps (30 seconds)

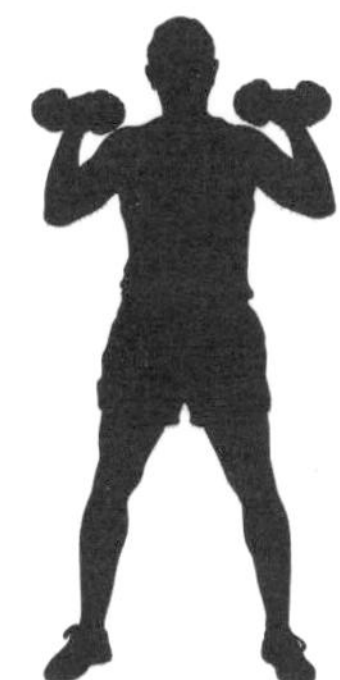

5-MINUTE ARMS WORKOUTS

ARMS 1

- Dumbbell Shoulder Press (30 seconds)
- Dumbbell Biceps Curls (30 seconds)
- Dumbbell Triceps Kickbacks (30 seconds)
- Dumbbell Side Raises (30 seconds)
- Dumbbell Front Raises (30 seconds)

ARMS 2

- Dumbbell Jabs (30 seconds)
- Dumbbell Biceps Curls (30 seconds)
- Dumbbell Triceps Kickbacks (30 seconds)
- Dumbbell Uppercuts (30 seconds)
- One-Dumbbell Overhead Extension (30 seconds)

ARMS 3

- Dumbbell Biceps Curls (60 seconds)
- Dumbbell Triceps Kickbacks (60 seconds)
- Dumbbell Front and Side Raises (30 seconds)

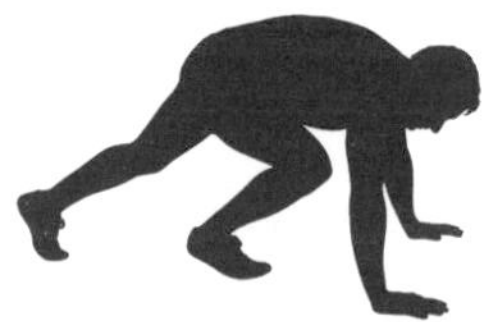

5-MINUTE CARDIO WORKOUTS

CARDIO 1

- Running in Place (75 seconds)
- Jumping Jacks (75 seconds)

CARDIO 2

- Running in Place (60 seconds)
- Jumping Jacks (30 seconds)
- Skaters (30 seconds)
- Pop Squats (30 seconds)

CARDIO 3

- Jumping Jacks (60 seconds)
- Jump Lunges (30 seconds)
- Mountain Climbers (30 seconds)
- Burpees (30 seconds)

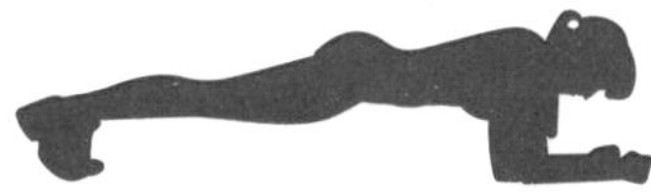

5-MINUTE CORE WORKOUTS

CORE 1

- Hand Crunches (30 seconds)
- Bridge (30 seconds)
- Back Stretch 1 (15 seconds each side)
- Hand Crunches (30 seconds)
- Bridge (30 seconds)

CORE 2

- Straight-Arm Plank (30 seconds)
- Bent-Knee Oblique (30 seconds each side)
- Double Crunch (30 seconds)
- Bridge Alternating Foot (30 seconds)

CORE 3

- Four-Point Alternating Plank (30 seconds)
- Side Plank (30 seconds each side)
- Bicycle Crunch (30 seconds)
- Bent-Arm Plank (30 seconds)

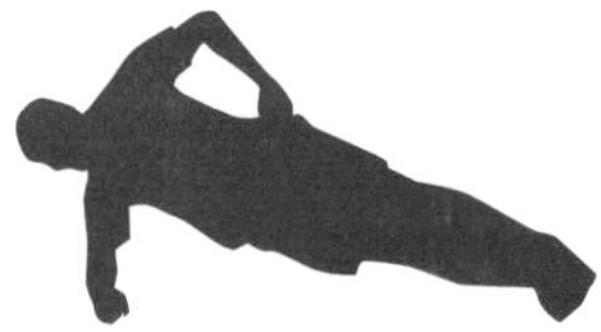

5-MINUTE LOWER BACK WORKOUTS

LOWER BACK 1

- Swimmer (60 seconds)
- Child's Pose Stretch (15 seconds)
- Bird Dog (60 seconds)
- Child's Pose Stretch (15 seconds)

LOWER BACK 2

- Superman (60 seconds)
- Cat-Cow Stretch (15 seconds)
- Seal (60 seconds)
- Cat-Cow Stretch (15 seconds)

LOWER BACK 3

- Bent-Arm Plank (60 seconds)
- Child's Pose Stretch (15 seconds)
- Side Plank (30 seconds each side)
- Child's Pose Stretch (15 seconds)

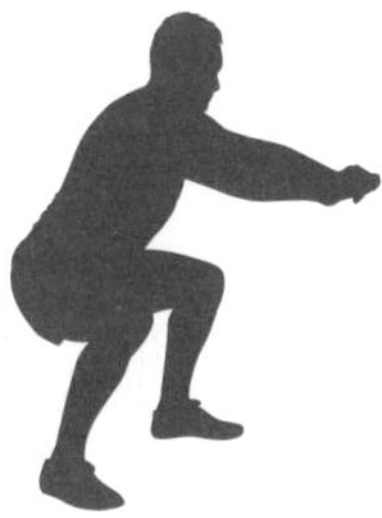

5-MINUTE LOWER BODY WORKOUTS

LOWER BODY 1

- Squats (30 seconds)
- Stationary Lunge (30 seconds each side)
- One-Leg Floor Touch (15 seconds each side)
- Standing Calf Raises (30 seconds)

LOWER BODY 2

- Alternating Forward Lunge (30 seconds)
- Alternating Back Lunge (30 seconds)
- Alternating Side Lunges (30 seconds)
- One-Leg Dumbbell Deadlift (30 seconds each side)

LOWER BODY 3

- One-Leg Stand Up (30 seconds each side)
- Step Up (30 seconds each side)
- Box Jumps (30 seconds)

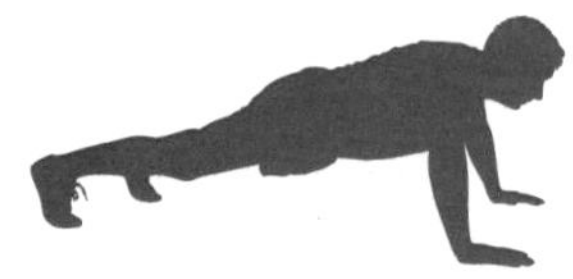

5-MINUTE Rx WORKOUTS

SHOULDERS RX

- Scarecrow Rotation (30 seconds)
- External Rotation (30 seconds)
- Internal Rotation (30 seconds)
- External Rotation (30 seconds)
- Internal Rotation (30 seconds)

LOWER BACK RX

- Bird Dog (30 seconds)
- Swimmer (30 seconds)
- Back Stretch 1 (15 seconds each side)
- Seal (30 seconds)
- Plank (30 seconds)

KNEE RX

- Stationary Lunge (30 seconds each side)
- Step Ups (30 seconds each side)
- Squats (30 seconds)

5-MINUTE STRETCHES

STRETCH: TOTAL BODY

- Standing Quad (15 seconds each side)
- Standing Glute (15 seconds each side)
- Kneeling Hamstring (15 seconds each side)
- Kneeling Hip Flexor (15 seconds each side)
- Kneeling Calf (15 seconds each side)
- Neck (15 seconds each side)
- Shoulder (15 seconds each side)
- Triceps (15 seconds each side)
- Back Stretch 1, 2, or 3 (15 seconds each side)
- Cat-Cow Stretch (15 seconds)
- Child's Pose (15 seconds)

STRETCH: LOW BACK

- Cat-Cow Stretch (30 seconds)
- Back Stretch 1 (30 seconds each side)
- Back Stretch 2 (30 seconds each side)
- Back Stretch 3 (30 seconds each side)
- Low Back Rotation (30 seconds each side)
- Child's Pose (30 seconds)

STRETCH: LOWER BODY

- Standing Quad (30 seconds each side)
- Kneeling Hamstring (30 seconds each side)
- Standing Glute (30 seconds each side)
- Side Quad (30 seconds each side)
- Kneeling Hip Flexor (30 seconds each side)

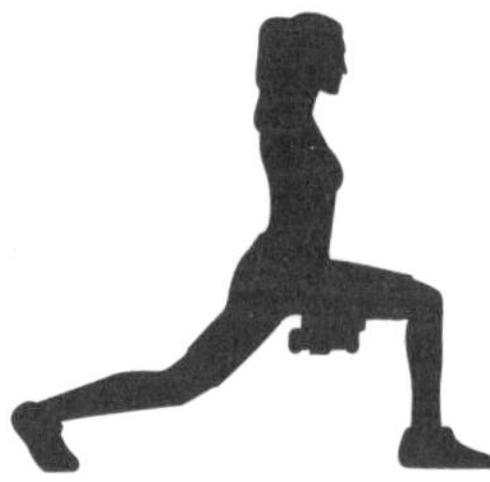

5-MINUTE TOTAL BODY WORKOUTS

TOTAL BODY 1

- Running in Place (30 seconds)
- Regular Push-ups (30 seconds)
- Squats (30 seconds)
- Jumping Jacks (30 seconds)
- Straight-Arm Plank (30 seconds)

TOTAL BODY 2

- Skaters (30 seconds)
- Alternating Front Lunge/Dumbbell Biceps Curls (30 seconds)
- Alternating Back Lunge/Dumbbell Shoulder Press (30 seconds)
- Regular Push-ups with Alternating Raised Leg (30 seconds)
- Bicycle Crunches (30 seconds)

TOTAL BODY 3

- Burpees (30 seconds)
- Regular Push-up/Dumbbell Row Combo (30 seconds)
- Pop Squats (30 seconds)
- Double Crunch (30 seconds)
- Dumbbell Biceps Curls (30 seconds)

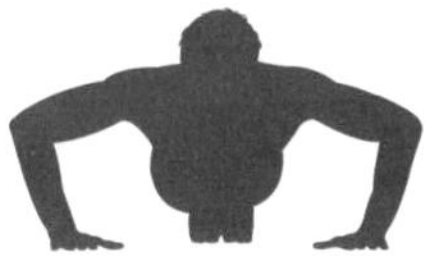

5-MINUTE UPPER BODY WORKOUTS

UPPER BODY 1

- Knee Push-ups (30 seconds)
- Dumbbell Rows (30 seconds)
- Dumbbell Shoulder Press (30 seconds)
- Dumbbell Biceps Curls (30 seconds)
- Dumbbell Triceps Kickbacks (30 seconds)

UPPER BODY 2

- Regular Push-ups (30 seconds)
- Dumbbell Bent-Arm Rows (30 seconds)
- Dumbbell Front and Side Raises (30 seconds)
- Dumbbell Biceps Curls (30 seconds)
- Dumbbell Jabs (30 seconds)

UPPER BODY 3

- Push-up/Dumbbell Row Combo (60 seconds)
- Dumbbell Biceps Curls/Dumbbell Shoulder Press Combo (60 seconds)
- One-Dumbbell Overhead Extension (30 seconds)

16

EXERCISE DESCRIPTIONS

Here are detailed instructions for all of the exercises contained in the thirty micro workouts. Remember that proper form is crucial for both maximizing results as well as minimizing the chance of injury. When using weights, be sure to select ones that are challenging for the last few repetitions without compromising your form.

ALTERNATING BACK LUNGE

Keeping your chest up and your knees behind your toes, step backward with your right leg until your right knee is a few inches off the floor. Hold for 1 second, step back, then repeat with your left leg.

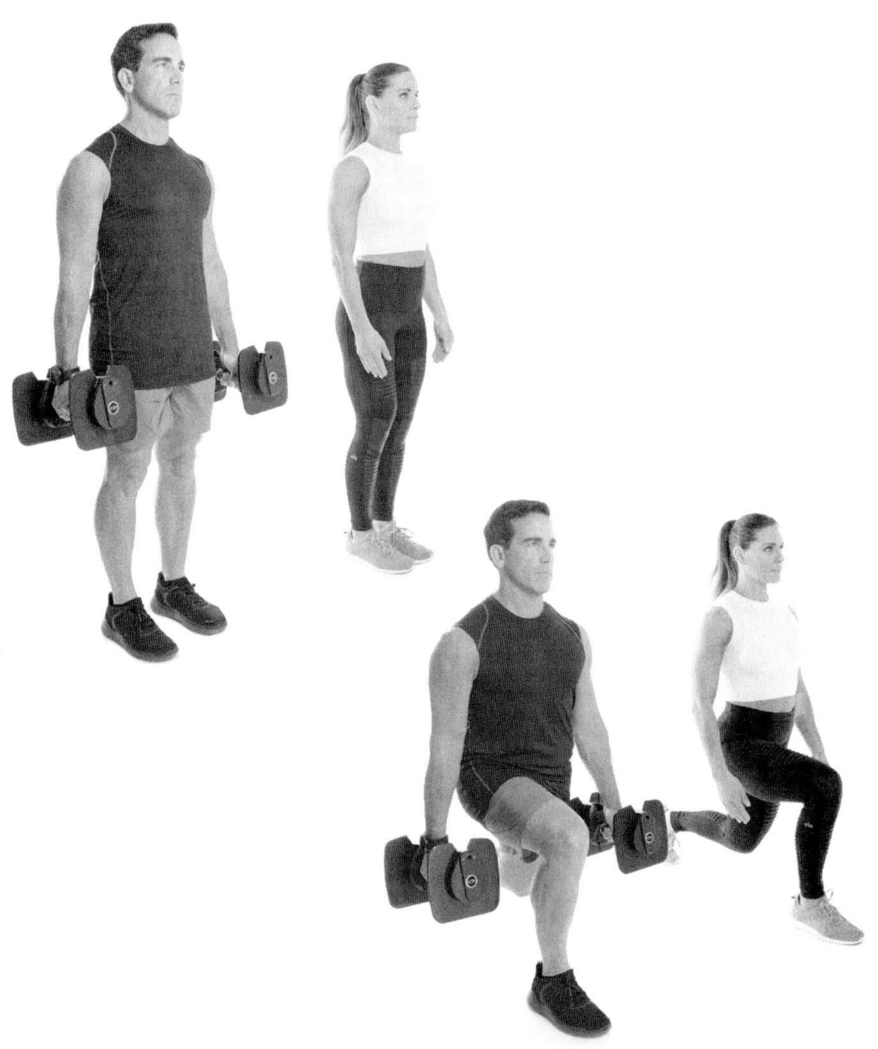

ALTERNATING BACK LUNGE/ SHOULDER PRESS

Stand with feet shoulder-width apart. Hold dumbbells in a goalpost position, with palms facing forward and arms bent 90 degrees. Keeping your chest up and your front knee behind your toes, slowly step forward with one leg until your back knee is a few inches off the ground while simultaneously pressing the weights up over your head until they are almost touching; then step back to starting position. Alternate legs.

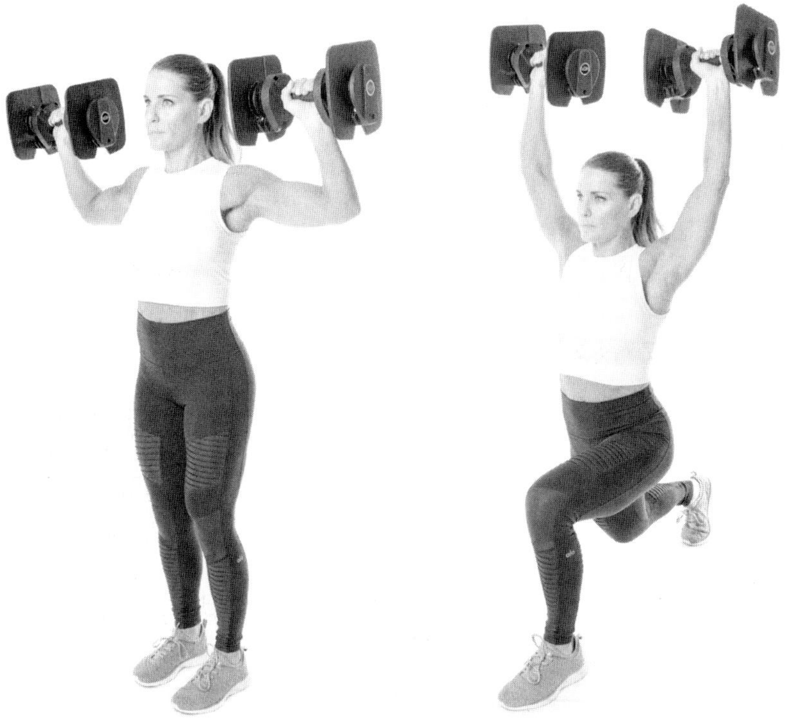

ALTERNATING FRONT LUNGE

Keeping your chest up and your knees behind your toes, step forward with your right leg until your left knee is a few inches off the floor. Hold for 1 second, step back, then repeat with your left leg.

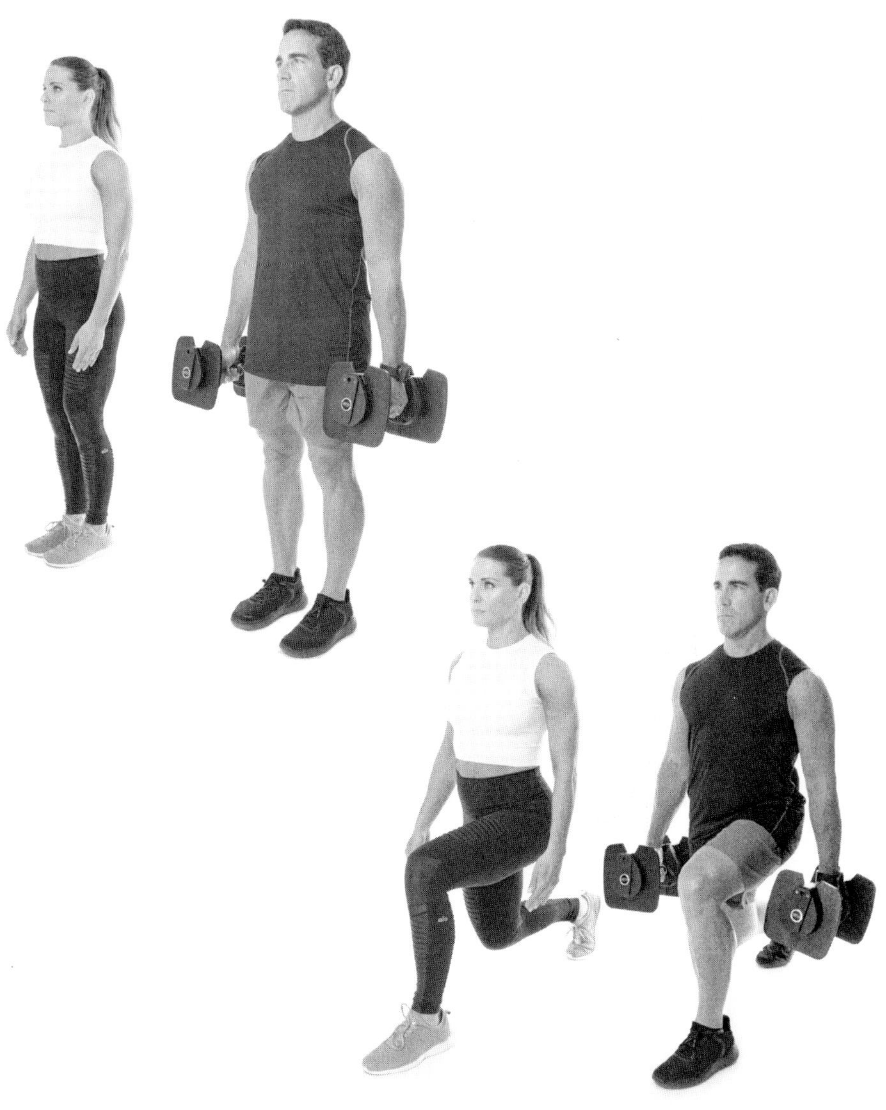

ALTERNATING FRONT LUNGE/ BICEPS CURLS

Stand with feet shoulder-width apart while holding dumbbells at your sides, palms facing away from you. Keeping your chest up and your front knee behind your toes, slowly step forward with one leg until your back knee is a few inches off the ground while simultaneously bending your elbows and bringing the weights up to your shoulders; then step back to starting position. Alternate legs.

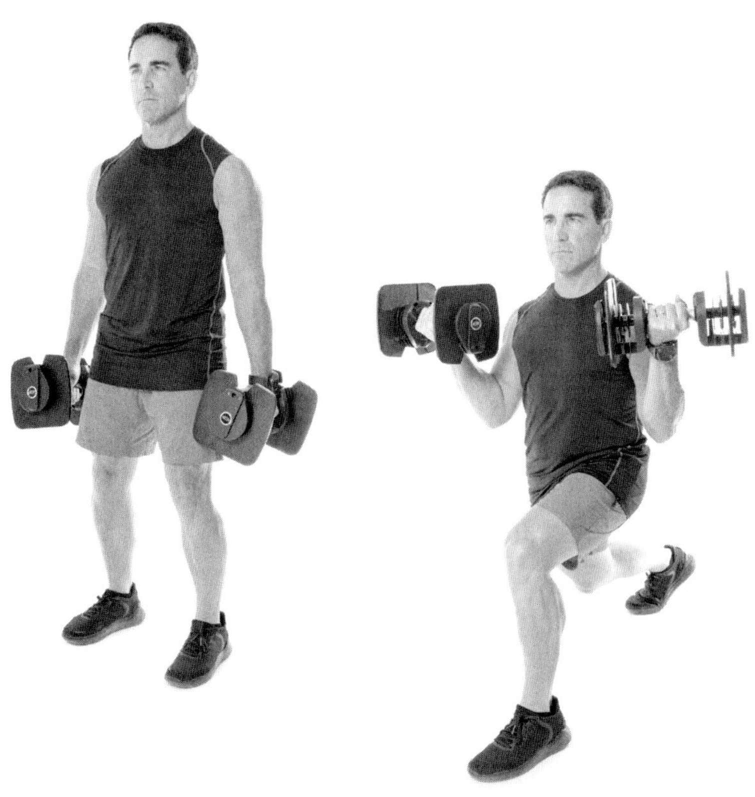

ALTERNATING SIDE LUNGE

Stand with feet shoulder-width apart while holding dumbbells at your sides, palms facing toward you. Keeping your chest up, slowly step to the right and bend your right knee, keeping your knee behind your toes and the weights on either side of your right shin, then step back to starting position. Alternate legs.

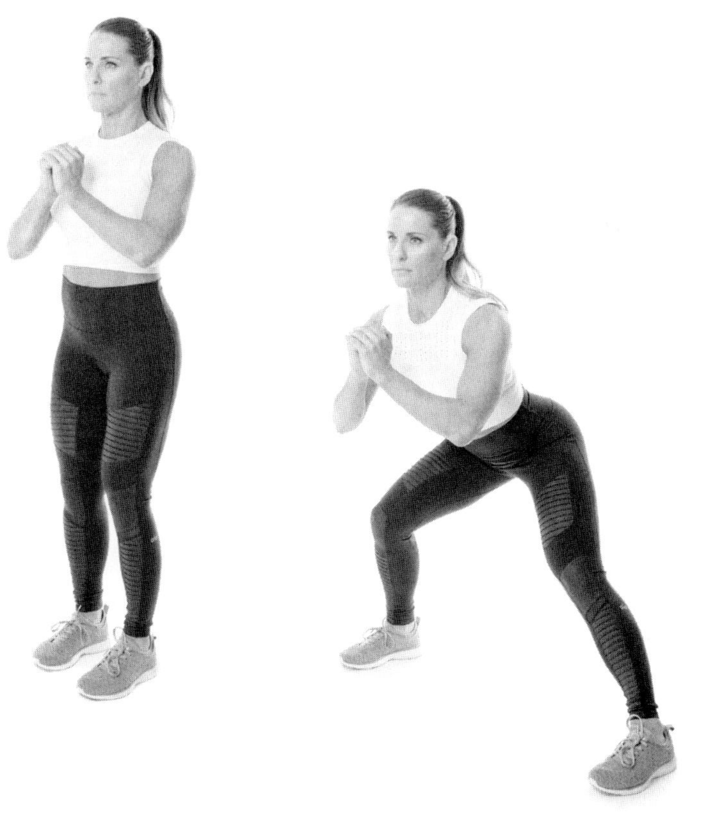

BACK STRETCH 1

Lie on your back with legs off the floor, knees pressed together and bent 90 degrees, arms straight out to your sides. Keeping them bent, slowly drop both legs to your left side, feeling a gentle stretch in your lower back. Repeat on the other side.

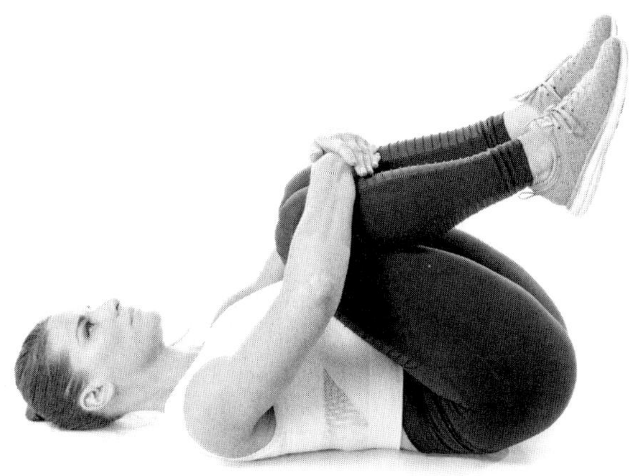

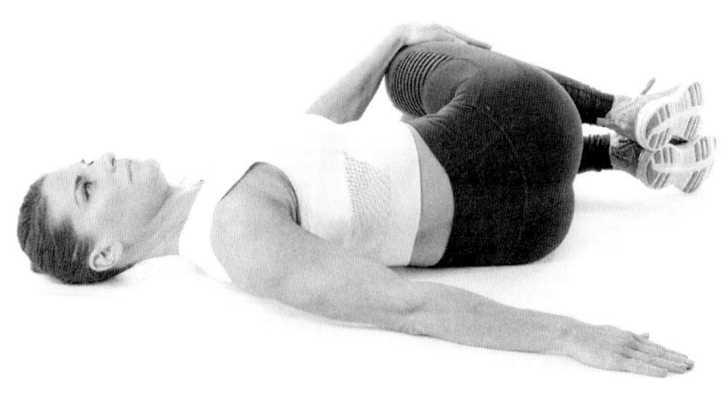

BACK STRETCH 2

Lie on your back with legs bent and off the floor, right leg crossed over your left, arms straight out to your sides. Keeping legs bent and shoulders on the floor, slowly drop both legs to your left side, feeling a gentle stretch in your lower back. Return to starting position, switch legs, and repeat on the other side.

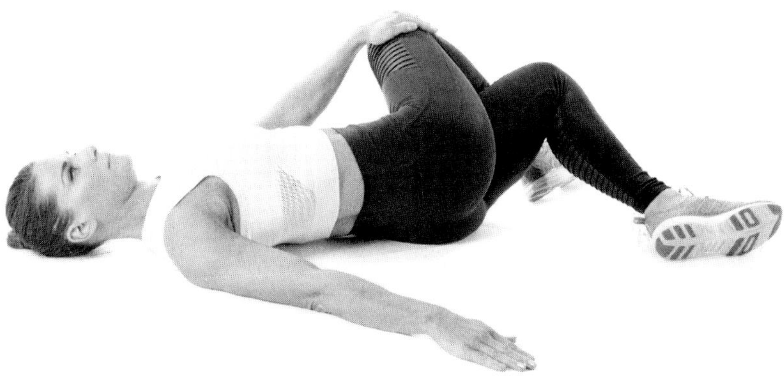

BACK STRETCH 3

Lie on your back with legs bent and off the floor, right leg crossed over your left, arms straight out to your sides. Keeping legs bent and shoulders on the floor, slowly drop both legs to your right side, feeling a gentle stretch in your lower back. Return to starting position, switch legs, and repeat on the other side.

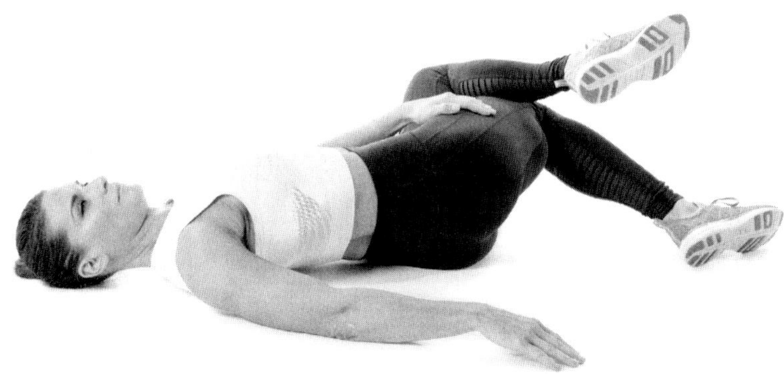

BENT-ARM PLANK

Assume a push-up position but support your upper body with your forearms, palms pressed to the floor. Keep your body perfectly straight and your abdominals pulled tight, but breathe normally.

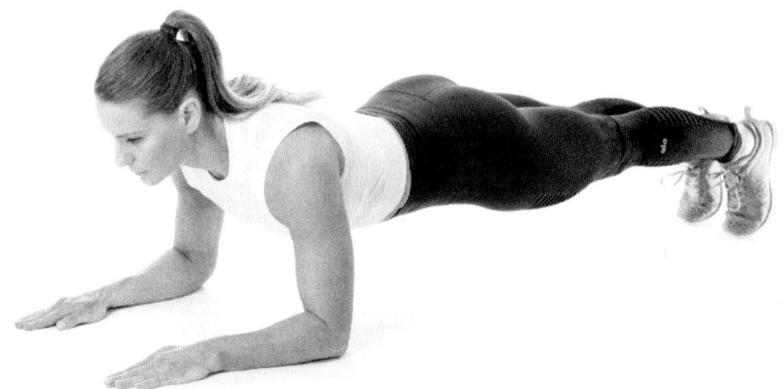

BENT-KNEE OBLIQUE CRUNCH

Lie on the floor with your right knee bent and your left leg crossed over, with the ankle resting on the thigh. Place your right hand behind your head, then bring the right elbow toward your raised foot while twisting and bringing the right shoulder blade up off the floor. Switch arms and legs and repeat on the other side.

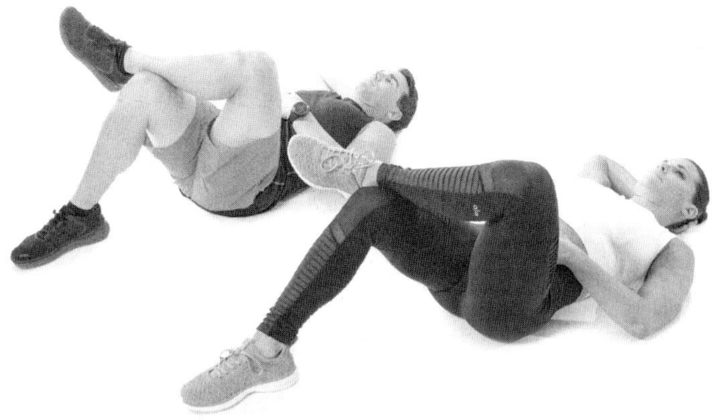

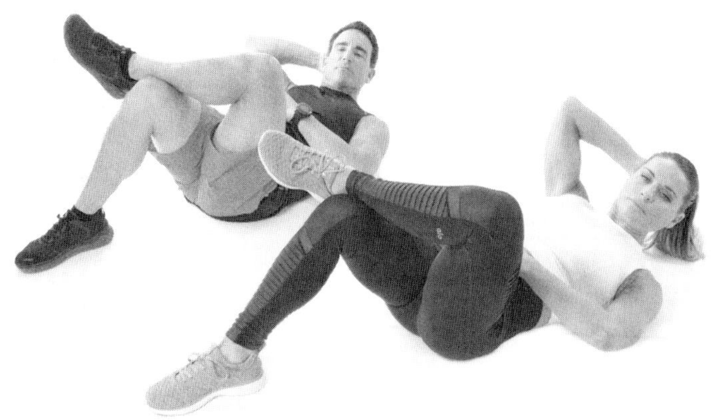

BICEPS CURLS/SHOULDER PRESS COMBO

Hold dumbbells with your elbows tucked in to your sides and your palms facing forward. Slowly raise the weights toward your shoulders, hold for 1 second, and slowly lower them. Then, moving your arms into a goalpost position, press the dumbbells over your head until the ends are almost touching. Slowly lower them back to the starting position.

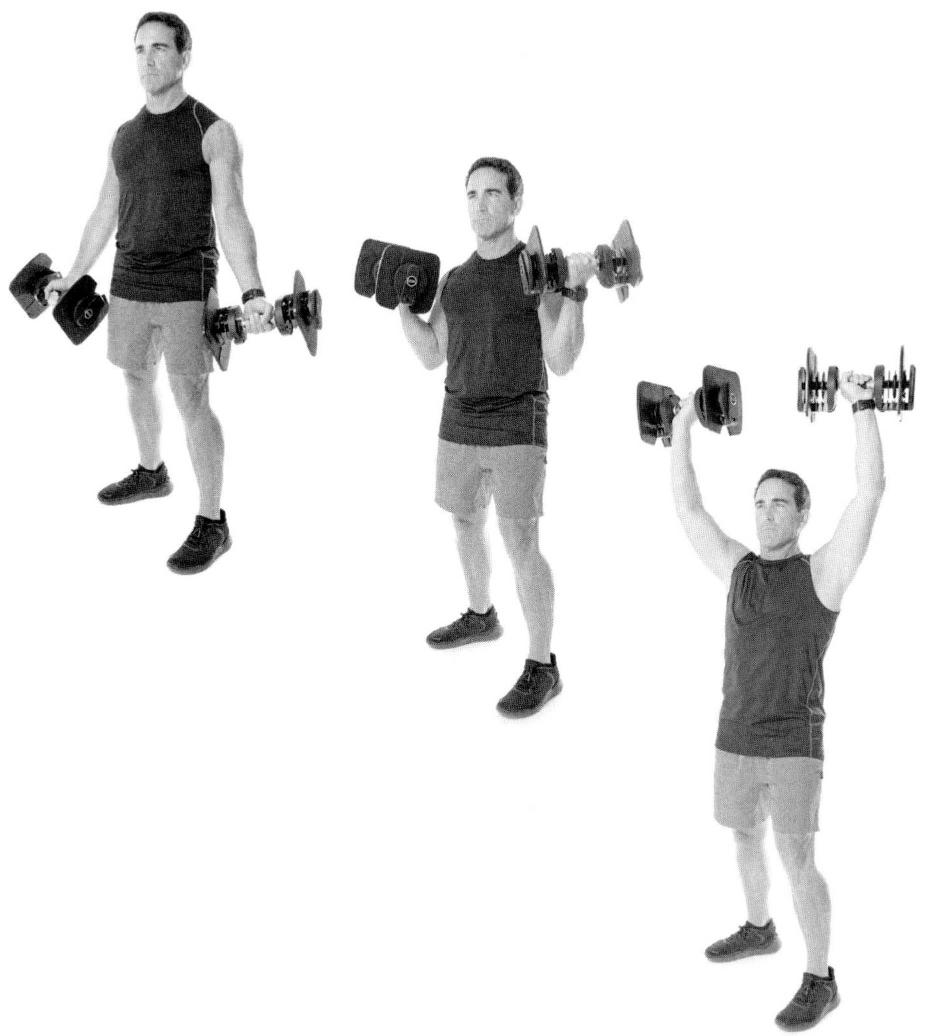

BICYCLE CRUNCH

Lying on your back with your hands behind your head, alternate bringing your right elbow to your left knee and your left elbow to your right knee. Keep your abdominals tight throughout.

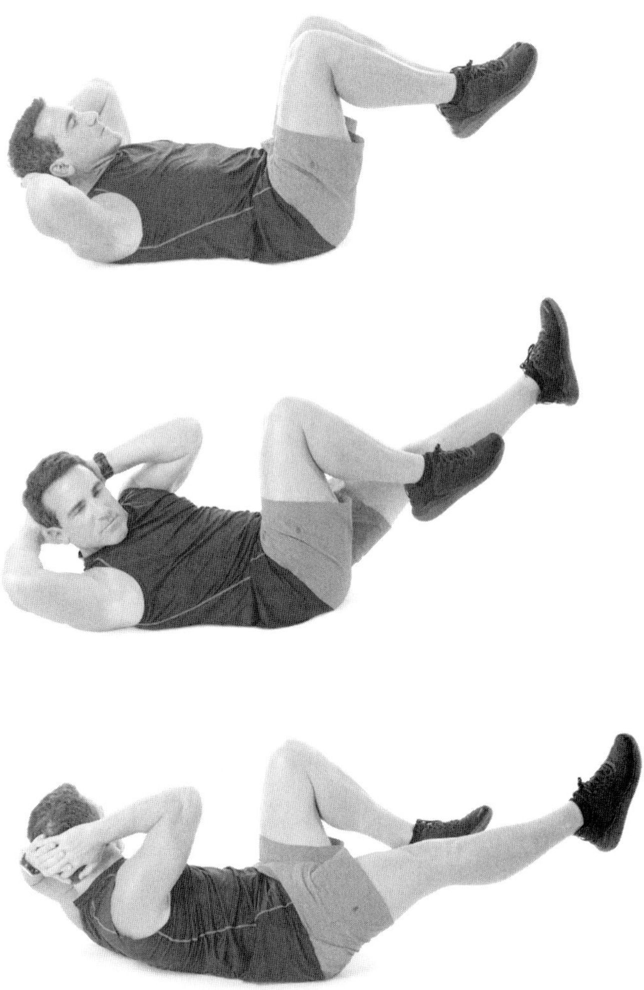

BIRD DOG

Kneeling on all fours, extend your left arm and right leg, hold for 1 second, and return to the starting position. Then extend your right arm and left leg, hold for 1 second, and return to the starting position.

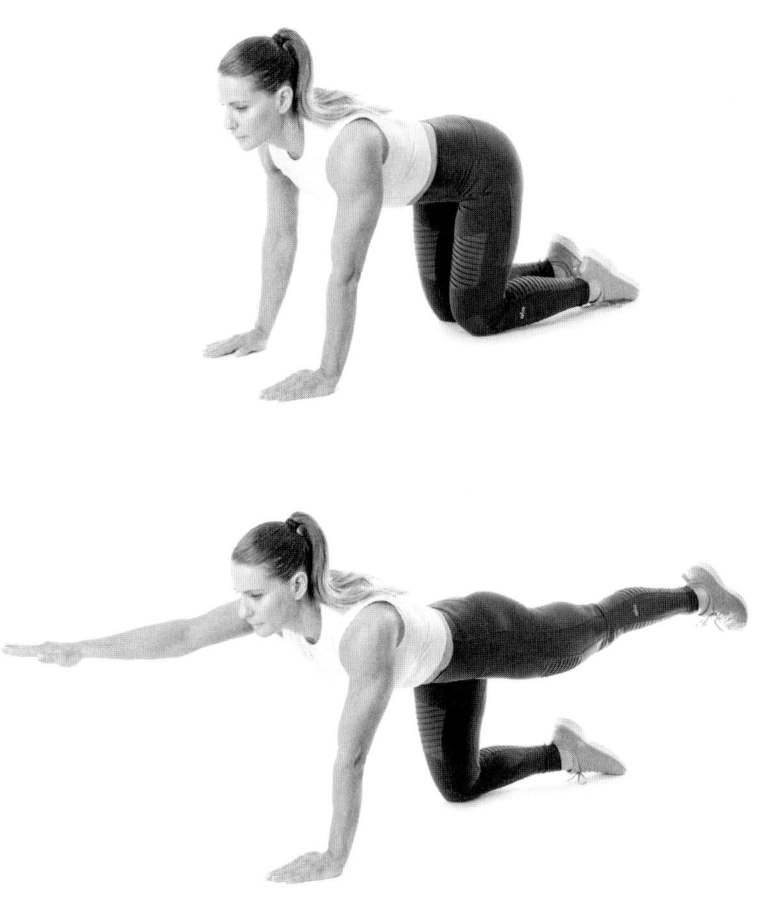

BOX JUMPS

Standing in front of a sturdy box roughly knee height, jump up onto it with both feet, landing as softly as possible; step back down and repeat.

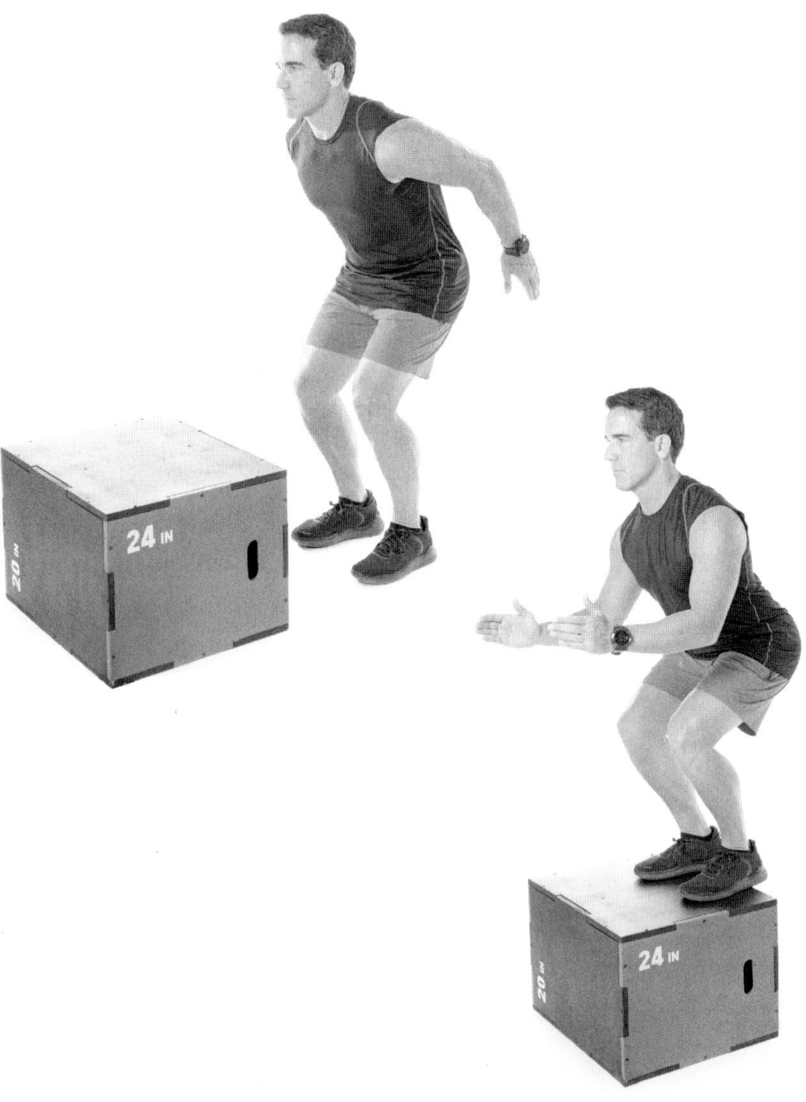

BRIDGE

Lie flat on your back with knees bent. Lift your body off the floor, forming a straight line and supporting yourself with your shoulders and your feet. Hold.

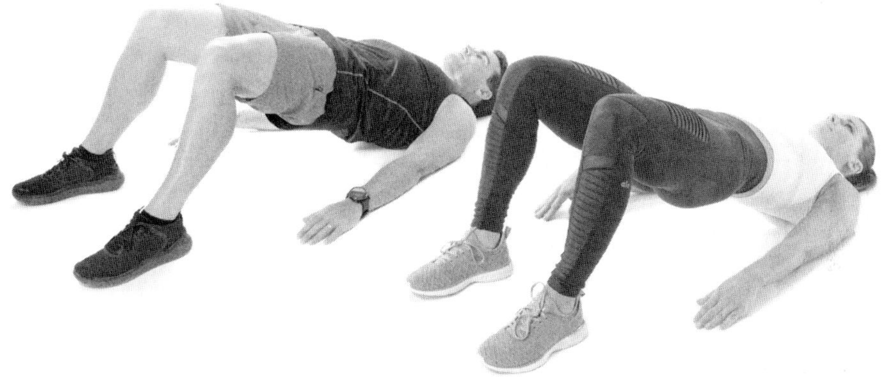

BRIDGE ALTERNATING FOOT

Lie flat on your back with knees bent. Lift your body off the floor, forming a straight line and supporting yourself with your shoulders and your feet. Lift one leg off the floor and straighten it in line with your body. Hold; then alternate legs.

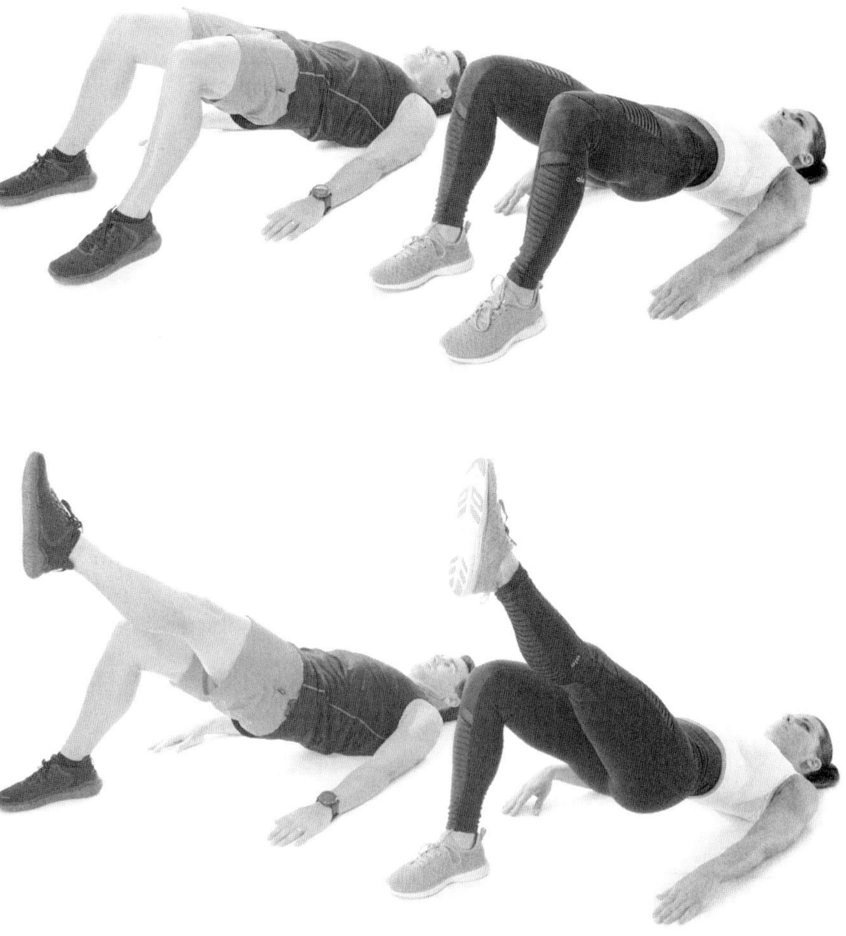

BULGARIAN SPLIT SQUAT

Stand in front of a bench or box in a lunge position, with one foot resting behind you on the bench. Keeping the knee of your supporting leg behind your toes, slowly lower your body down until the leg is bent to 90 degrees, then return to starting position.

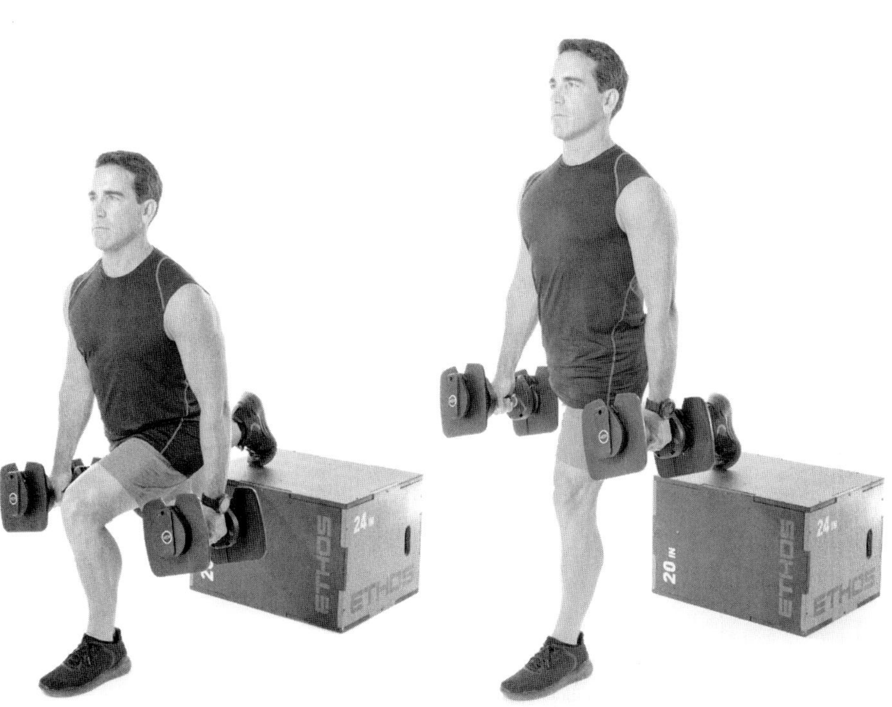

BURPEE

From a standing position, squat down and place your hands on the floor.

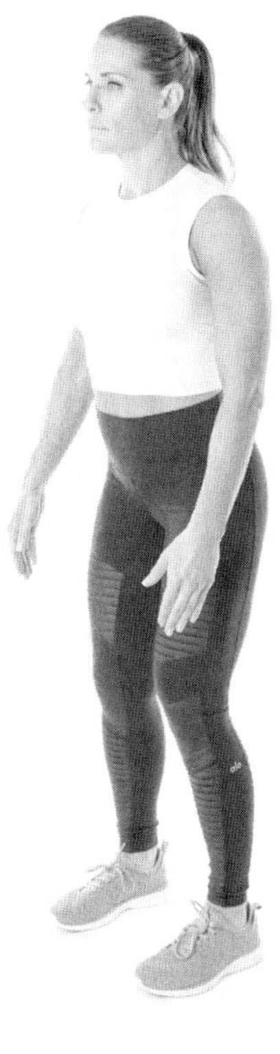

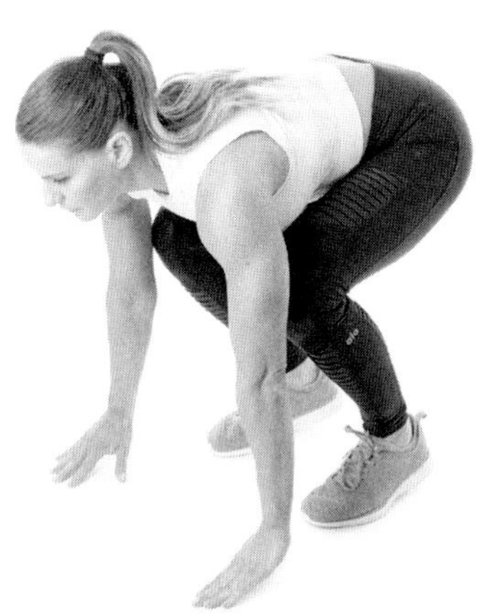

Kick or step both legs straight out behind you into a plank position, then jump back into a squat position. Stand and jump off the floor with arms overhead to complete the movement.

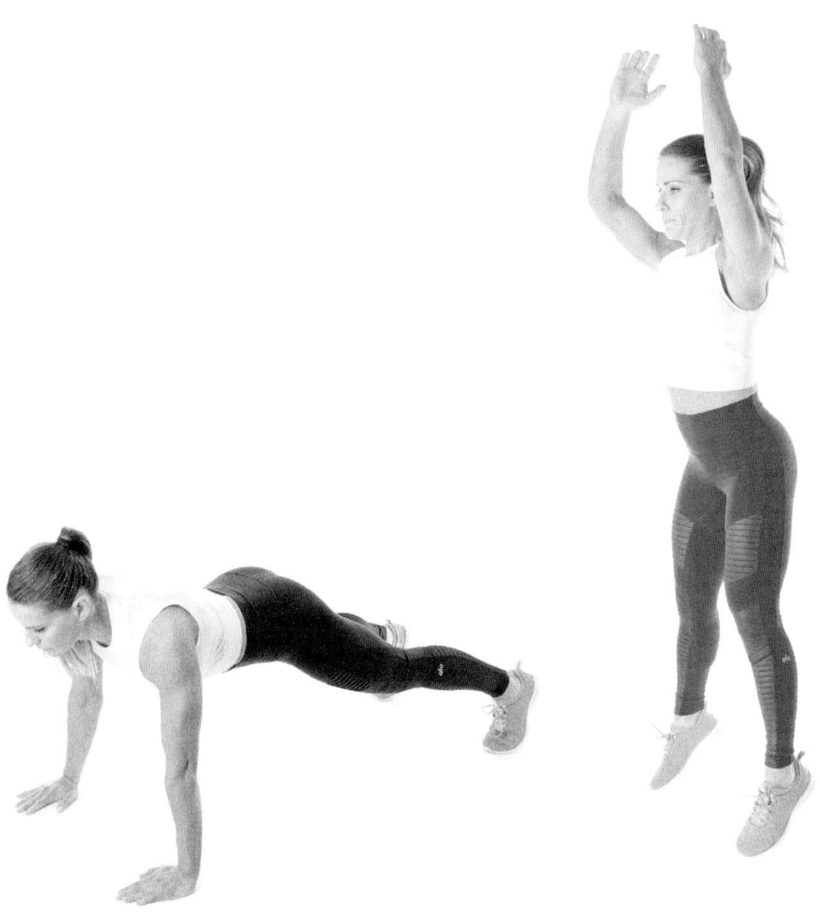

CAT-COW STRETCH

Kneeling on all fours, inhale while rounding your back and bringing your spine toward the ceiling and tucking your chin to your chest. Then exhale while pressing your bellybutton toward the floor and arching your head toward your back.

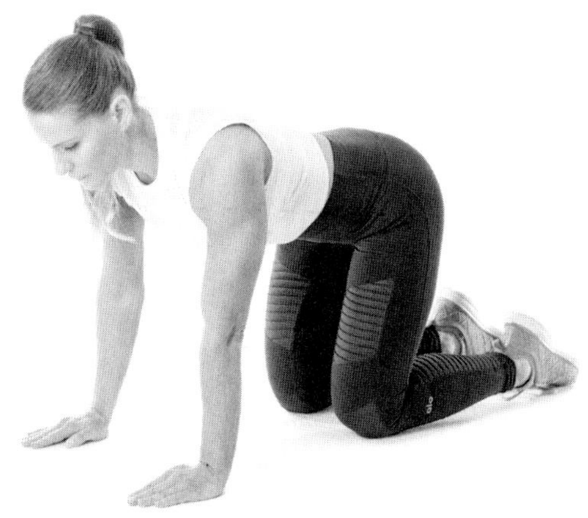

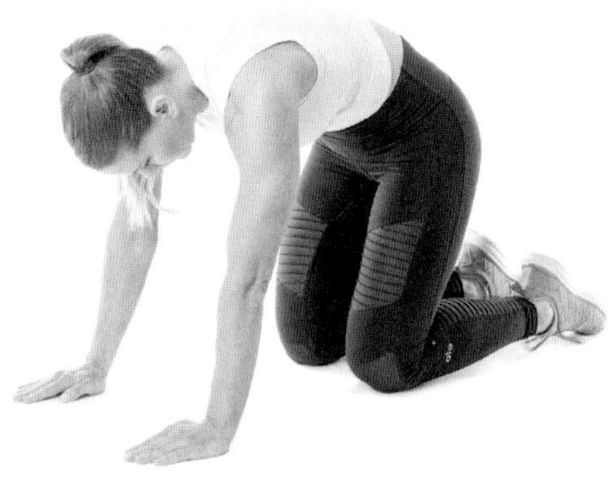

CHILD'S POSE STRETCH

Sitting with your legs tucked underneath you, reach forward on the floor in front of you, lengthening your spine.

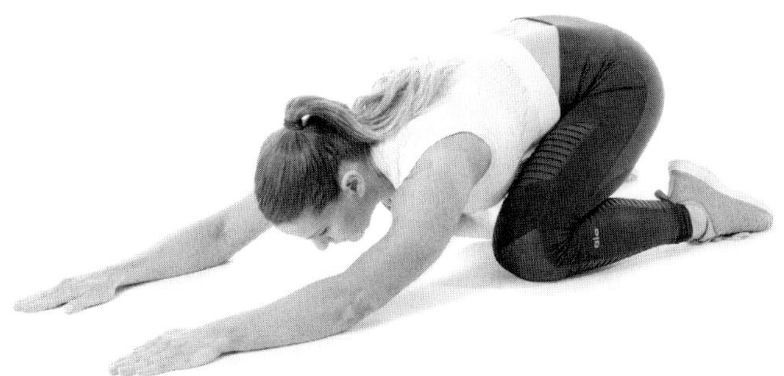

CROSS CRUNCH

Lie on the floor on your back, forming a letter X with your arms and legs. Keeping both straight, touch your right foot with left hand, return to starting position, then touch your left foot with your right hand.

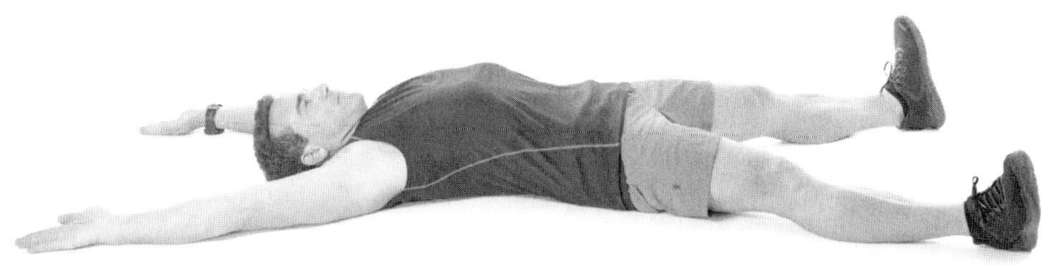

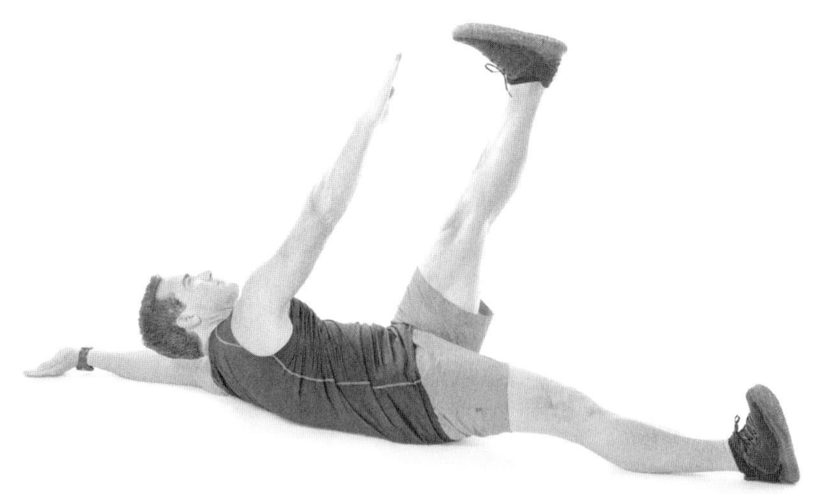

DOUBLE CRUNCH

Lie on your back with your legs raised in the air and your knees bent to 90 degrees. Making sure to keep your lower back pressed to the floor (a reverse pelvic tilt), extend your feet away from your body and pull them back toward your chest.

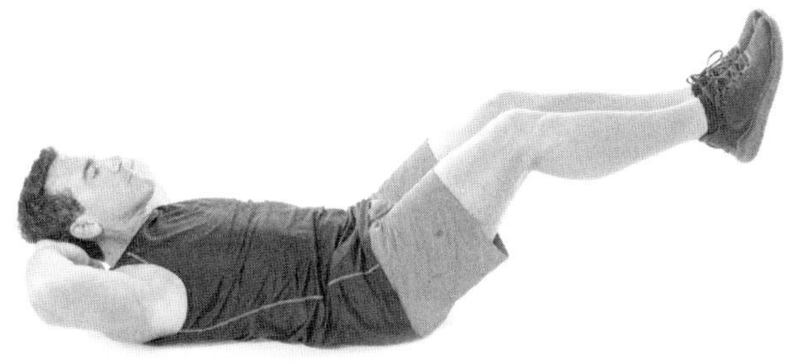

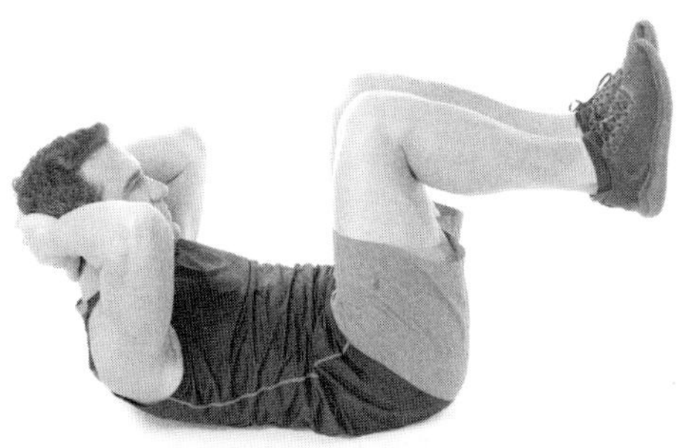

DUMBBELL BENT-ARM ROWS

Bend at the waist with your upper body as parallel as possible to the floor and your back flat, not rounded, holding dumbbells with palms facing behind you. Pull the weights up and out to the side until your arms are bent 90 degrees with your elbows level with your shoulders, then lower them back down to the starting position.

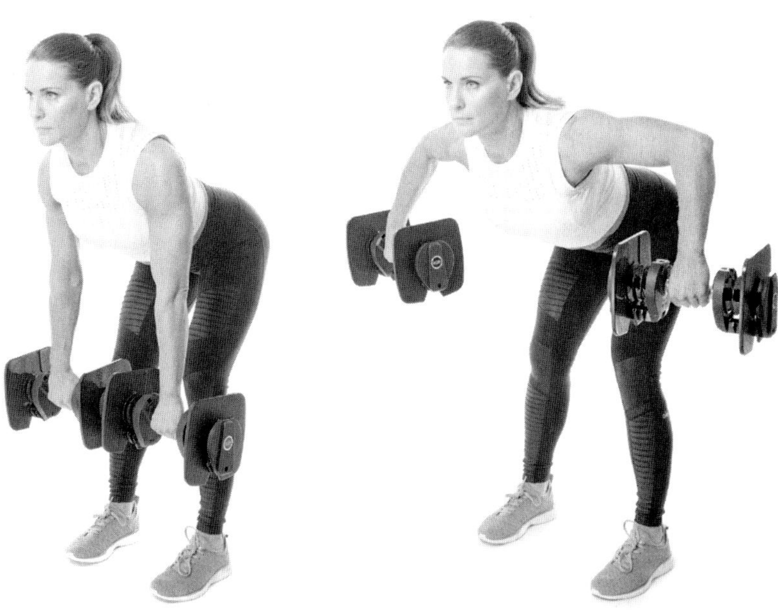

DUMBBELL BICEPS CURLS

Hold dumbbells with your elbows tucked in to your sides and your palms facing forward. Slowly raise the weights toward your shoulders, hold for 1 second, then slowly lower them.

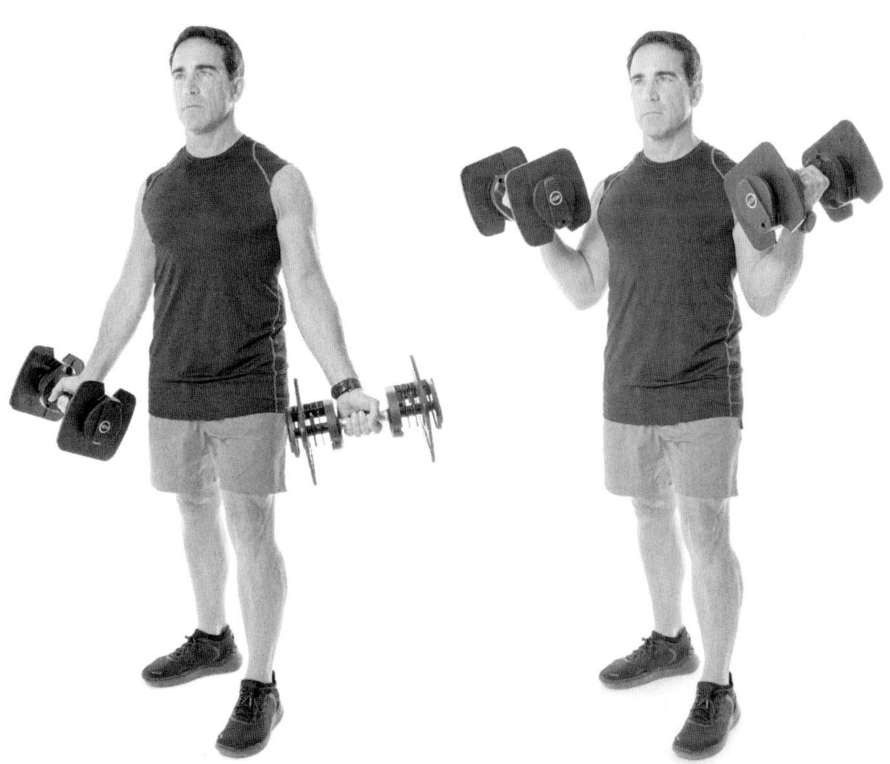

DUMBBELL FRONT AND SIDE RAISES

Stand in a split stance with one foot slightly in front of the other and knees slightly bent. Holding the dumbbells at your sides with elbows slightly bent, slowly raise them in front of you to shoulder height,

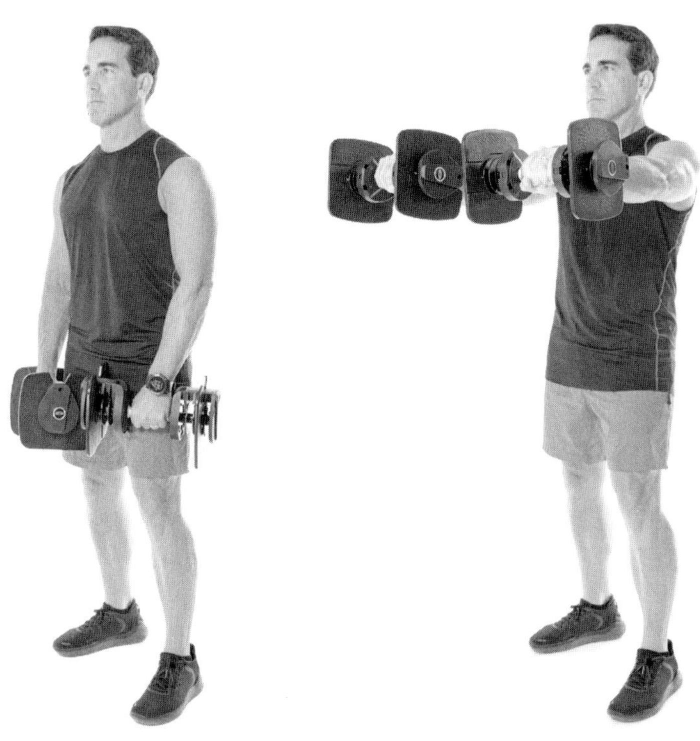

hold for 1 second, then slowly lower them. Next, slowly raise the weights out to your sides with your elbows slightly bent, up to shoulder height; hold for 1 second, then lower them to the starting position.

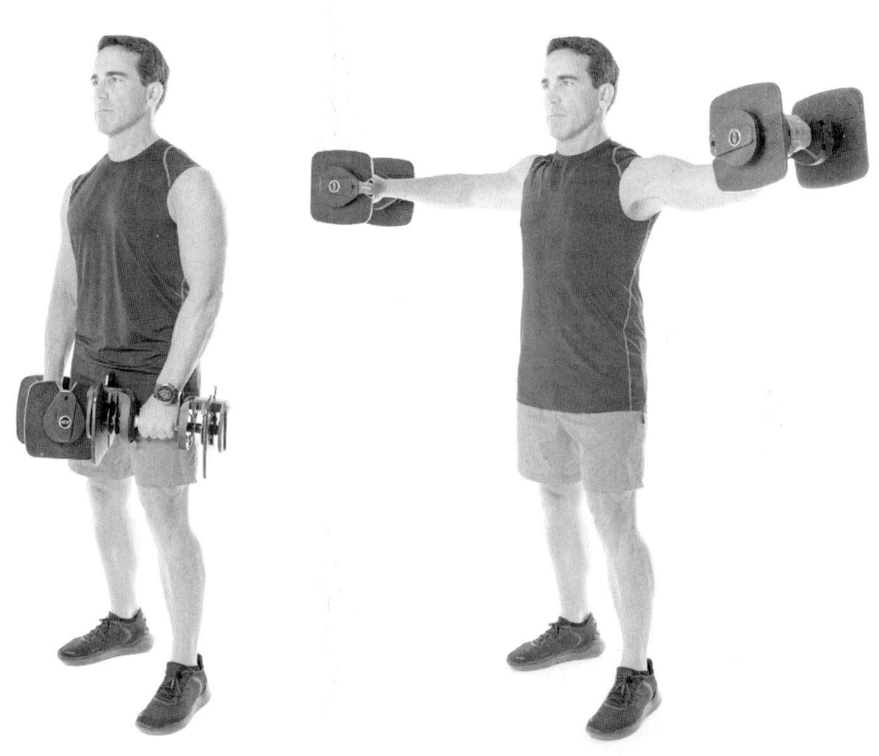

DUMBBELL FRONT RAISES

Stand holding dumbbells in front of your thighs. With elbows slightly bent, raise the weights in front of you up to shoulder height, then slowly lower them back to starting position.

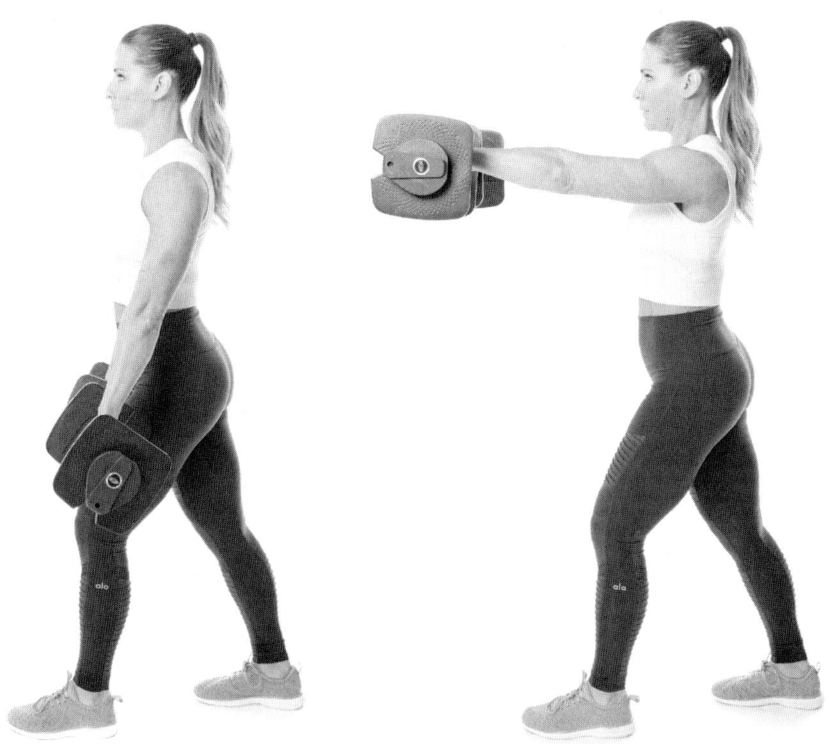

DUMBBELL JABS

Stand in a fighter's stance holding dumbbells in front of you. Extend one arm and punch straight ahead. Alternate arms.

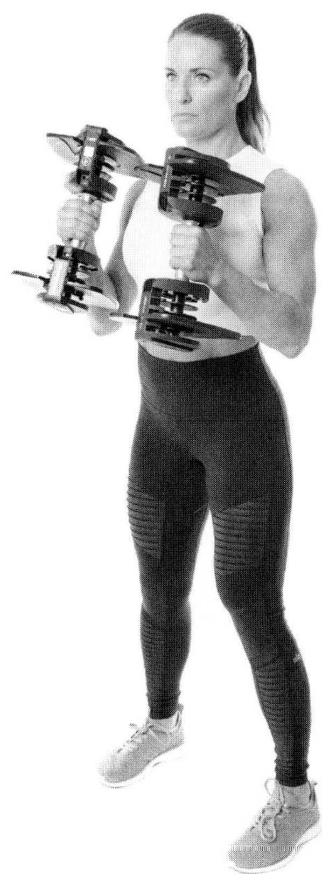

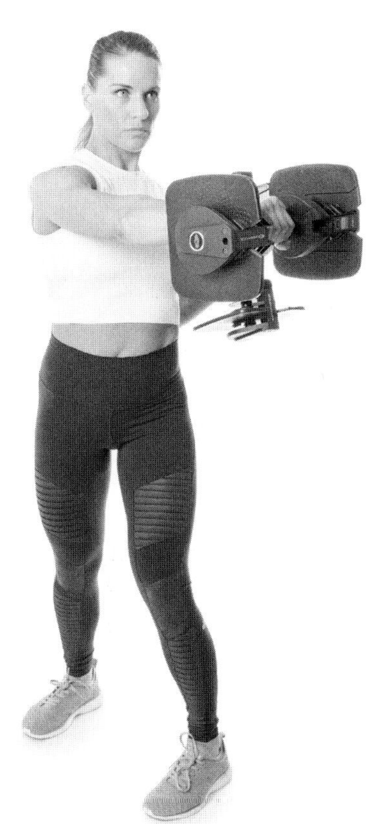

DUMBBELL ROWS

Bend at the waist with your upper body as parallel as possible to the floor and your back flat, not rounded. With your arms straight down and holding dumbbells facing one another, pull them up toward your body, hold for 1 second, then lower back down.

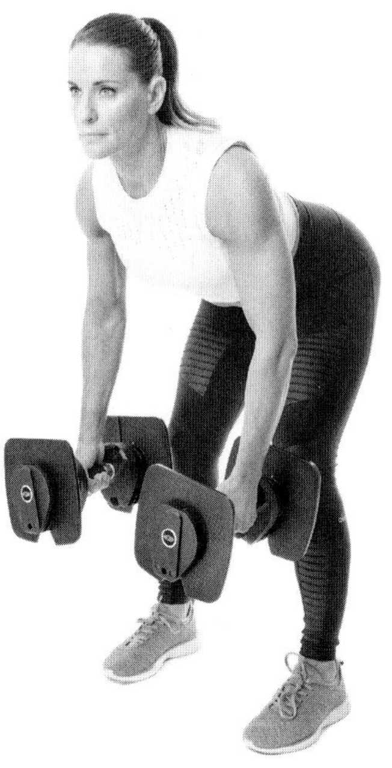

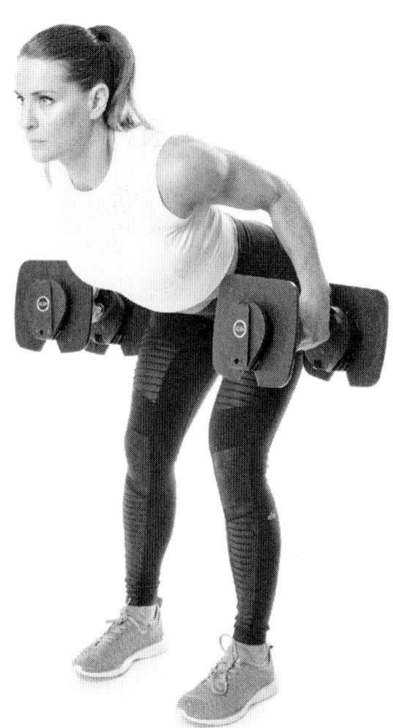

DUMBBELL SHOULDER PRESS

Stand while holding dumbbells in a goalpost position—with your elbows in line with your shoulders and your palms facing forward. Press the dumbbells over your head until the ends are almost touching, then slowly lower them to the starting position.

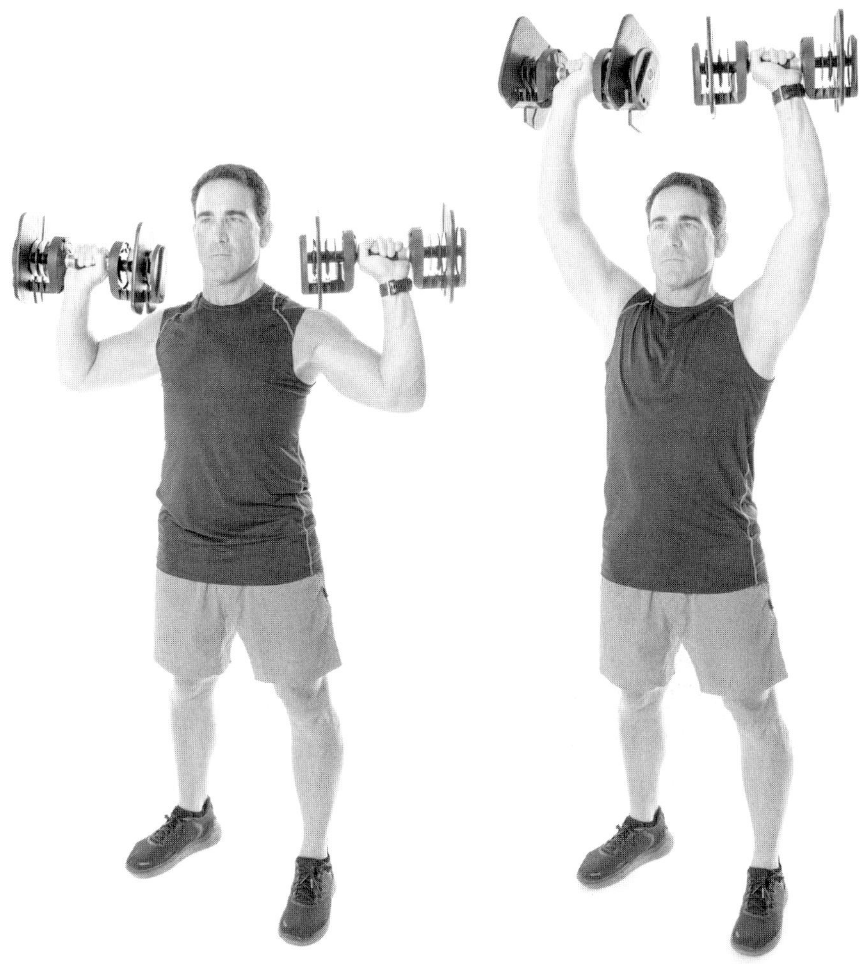

DUMBBELL SIDE RAISES

Stand holding dumbbells at your sides with palms facing front. With elbows slightly bent and pinned to your sides, raise the weights out to your sides up to shoulder height; then slowly lower them back to starting position.

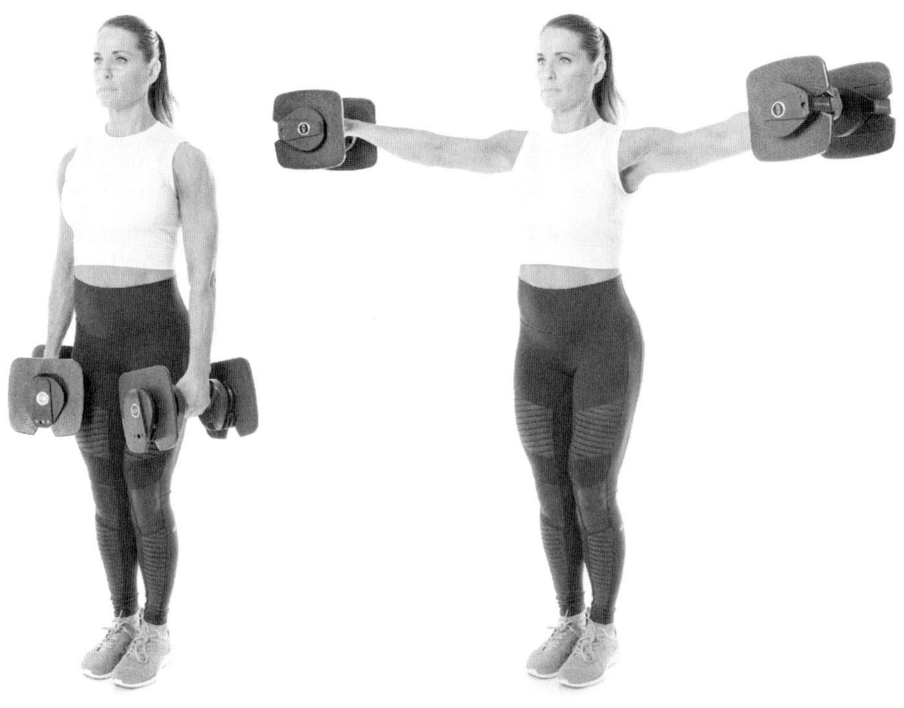

DUMBBELL TRICEPS KICKBACKS

Holding dumbbells, bend over until your upper body is as parallel to the floor as possible. Bring your elbows up so that your upper arms are parallel to the floor. With your palms facing toward you, extend the weights back and up until your arms are fully extended, hold for 1 second, then slowly lower them. Do not move your upper arms throughout the exercise.

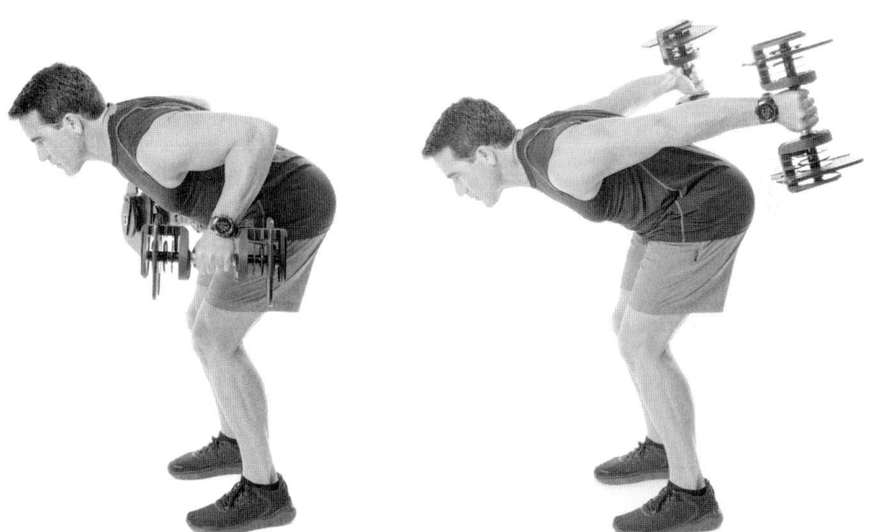

DUMBBELL UPPERCUTS

Stand holding dumbbells in front of you, arms bent 90 degrees and palms facing each other. Keeping your arm bent, punch the weight up in front of your chin with the palm facing you, then lower it back down to the starting position. Alternate arms.

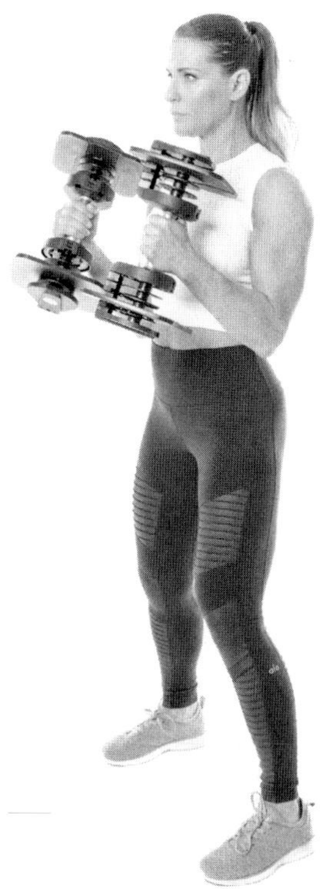

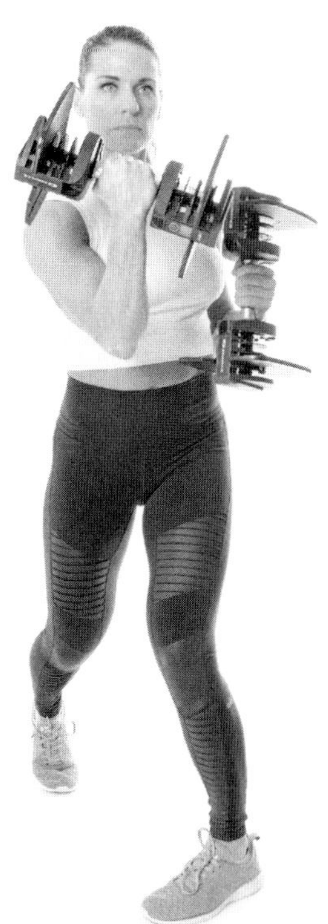

EXTERNAL ROTATION

Stand holding the handle of a resistance tube anchored to something stable, with your arm bent to 90 degrees and in front of you and your upper arm pressed against your body. Keeping your forearm parallel to the floor, pull the handle away from your body, hold for 1 second, then return to the starting position.

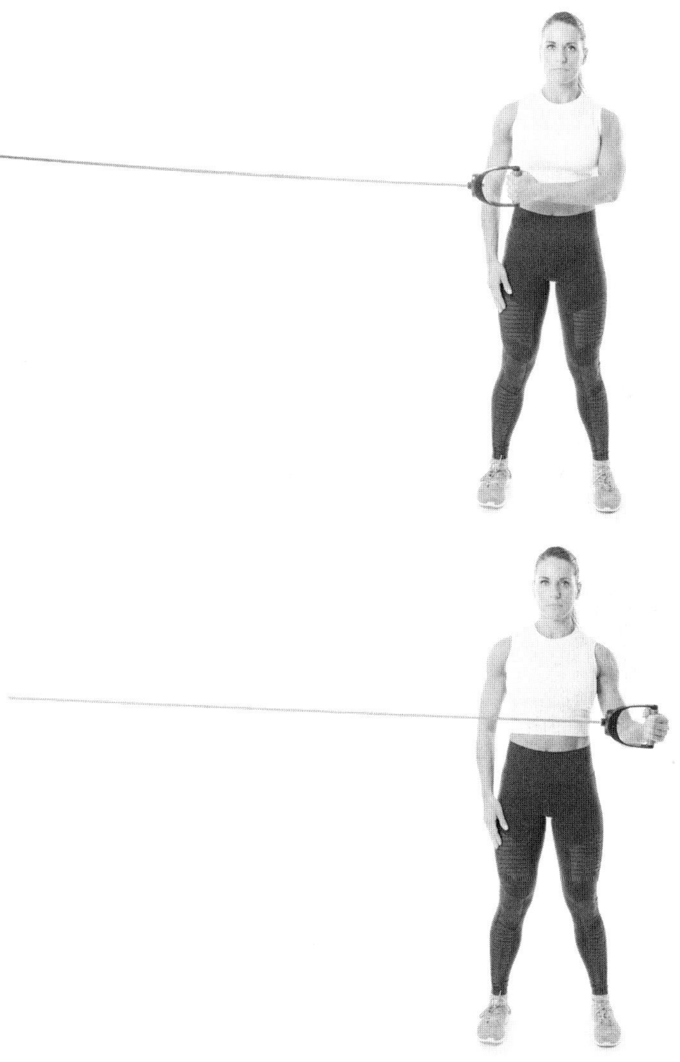

FOUR-POINT ALTERNATING PLANK

Hold your body at the top of a push-up position with your arms extended. Raise your right arm and left leg, hold for 1 second, and return to the starting position. Then raise your left arm and right leg, hold for 1 second, and return to the starting position.

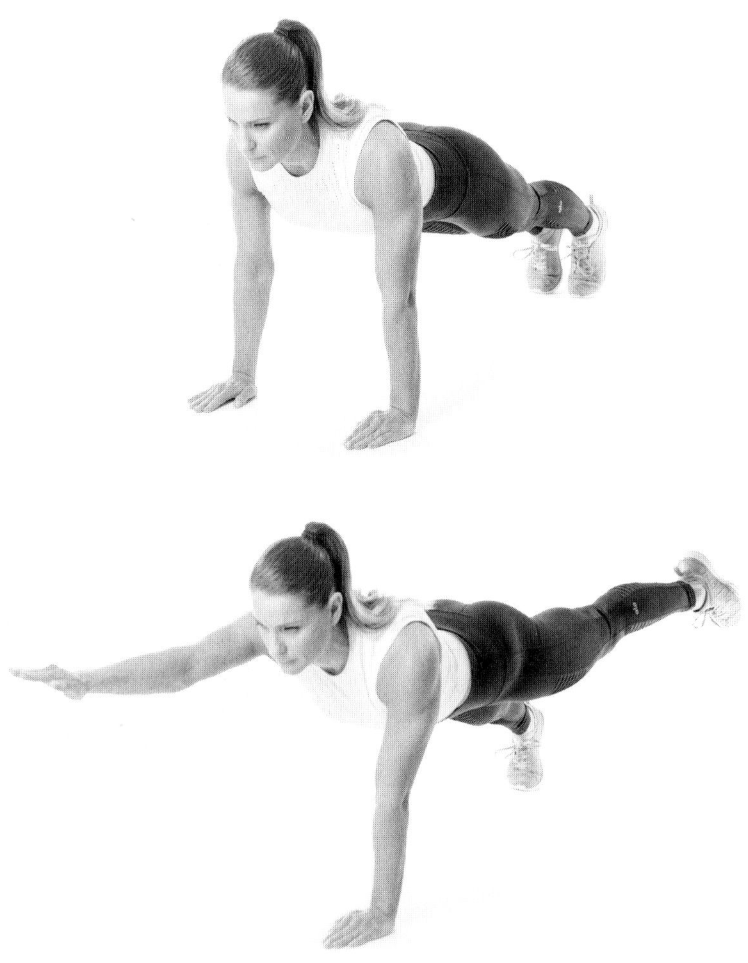

HAND CRUNCHES

Lie on your back with your knees bent, feet on the floor, and hands on your thighs. Lift your shoulders a few inches off the floor while sliding your hands toward your knees, keeping your chin off your chest, then lower back down.

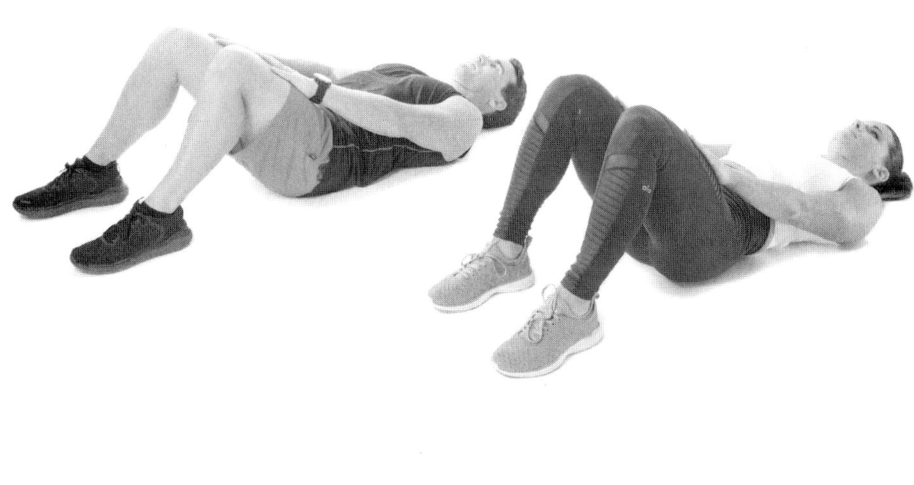

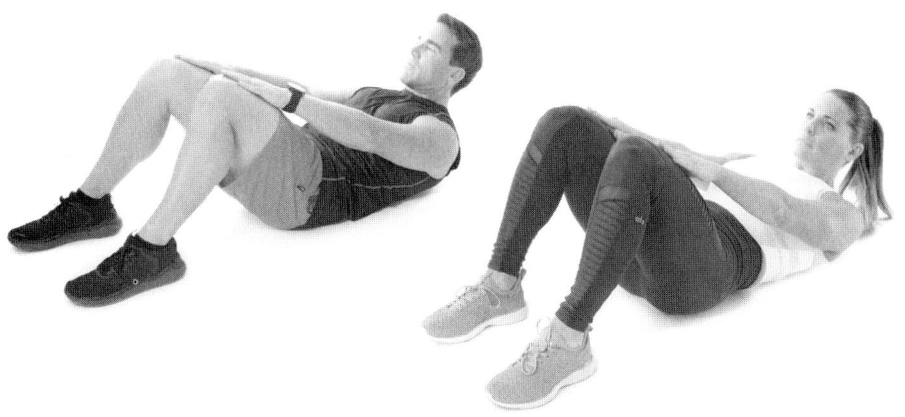

INTERNAL ROTATION

Stand holding the handle of a resistance tube anchored to something stable, with your arm bent to 90 degrees and to your side and your upper arm pressed against your body. Keeping your forearm parallel to the floor, pull the handle toward your body, hold for 1 second, then return to the starting position.

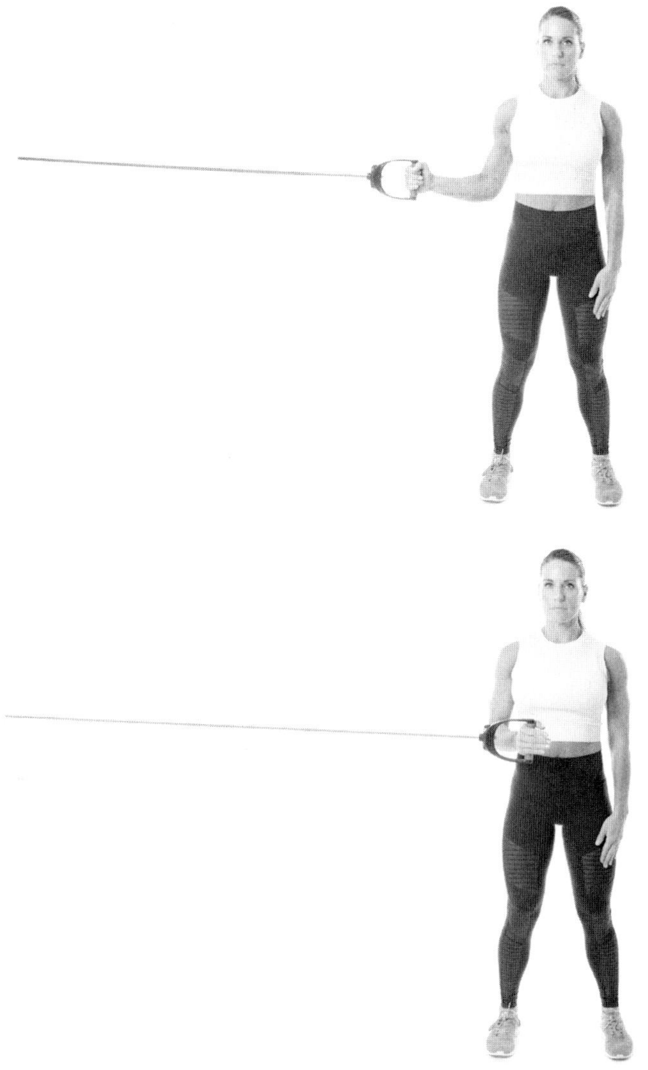

JABS

Stand in a fighter's stance, holding your hands in front of your chin. Extend one arm and punch straight ahead. Alternate arms.

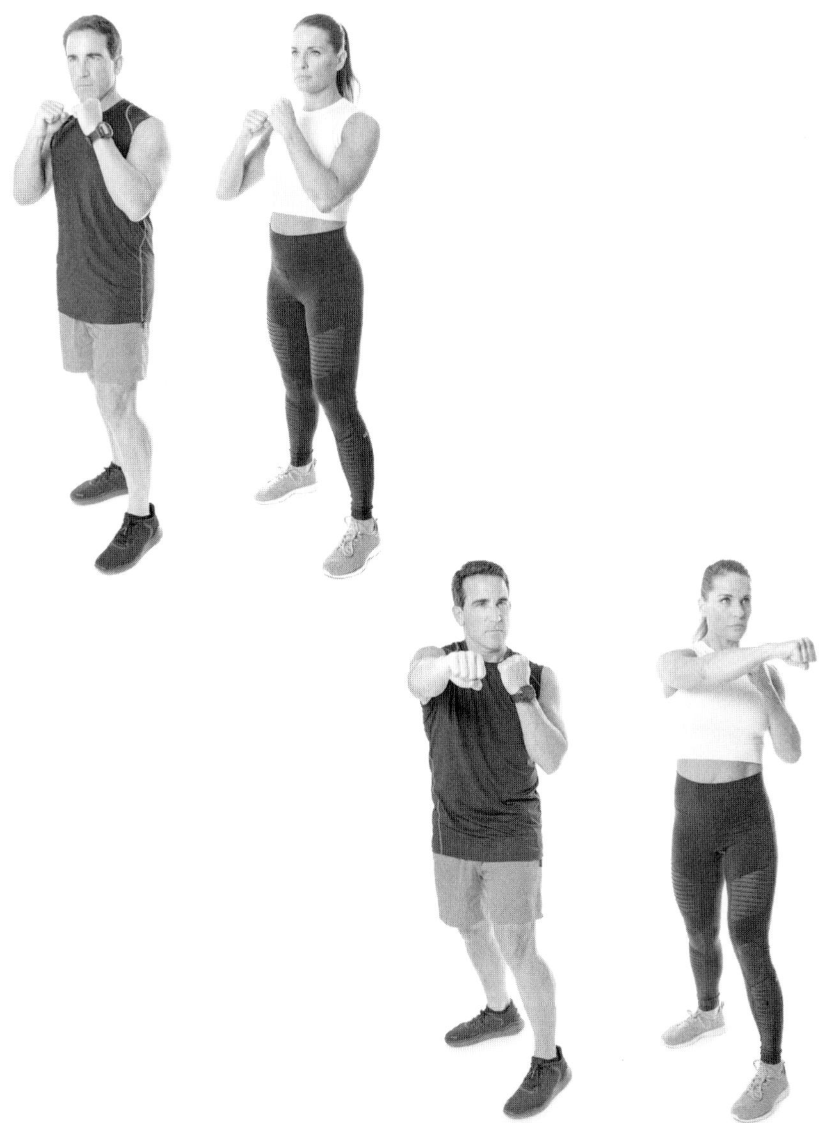

JUMP LUNGES

Stand in a split stance with your right foot forward and left foot back. Jump up and switch legs to land softly with your left foot forward and your right leg back.

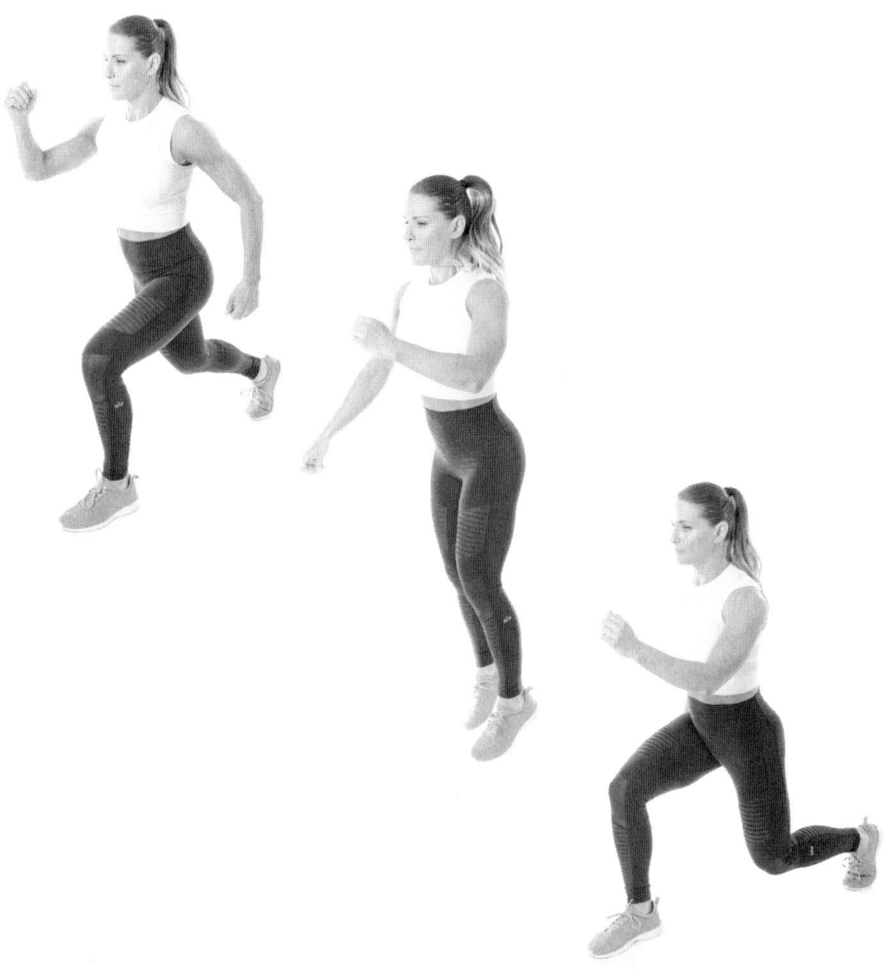

JUMPING JACKS

From a standing position, jump your feet a little wider than shoulder-width apart and bring your hands over your head, then jump back to starting position.

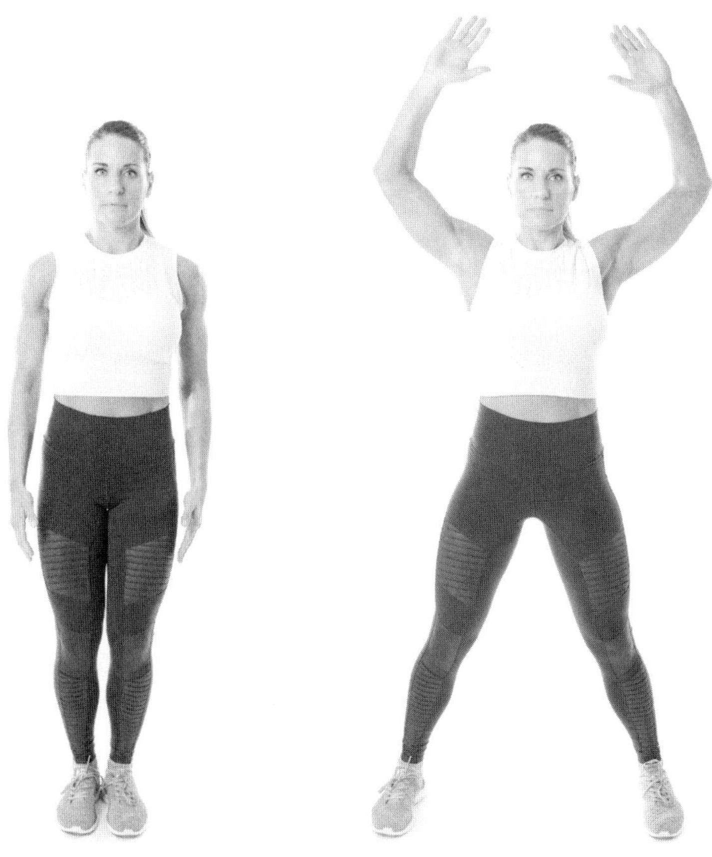

JUMPS

Standing with feet shoulder-width apart, jump up into the air while reaching with both hands over your head.

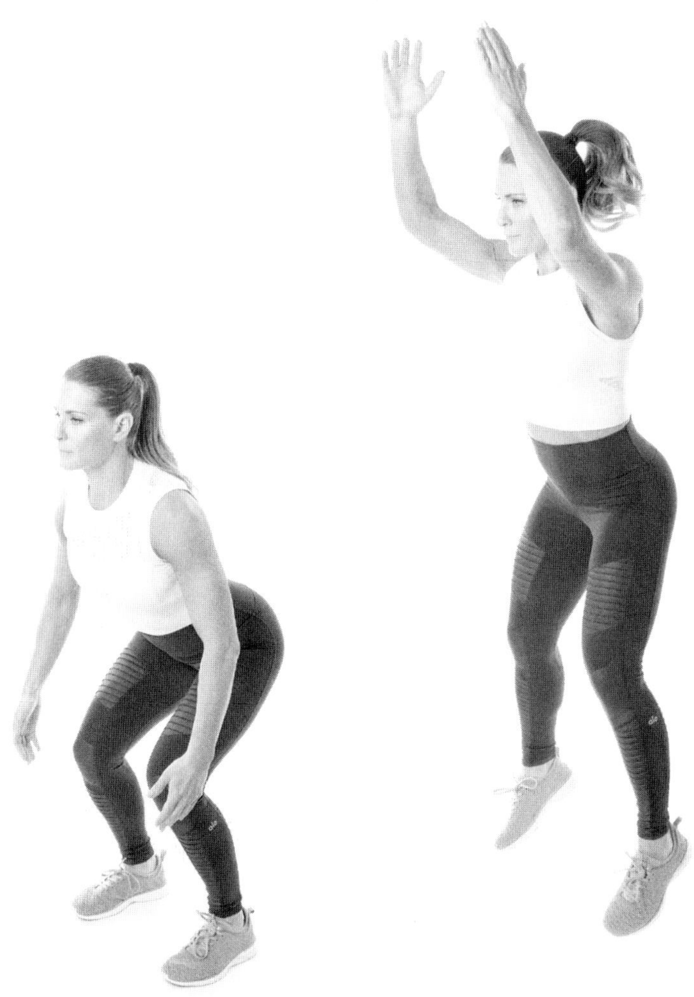

KNEE PUSH-UPS

Hold your body up off the floor in a straight line with your arms extended and a little wider than shoulder-width apart. Your knees and toes should touch the floor. Slowly bend your elbows until your chest is a few inches off the ground, then return to starting position.

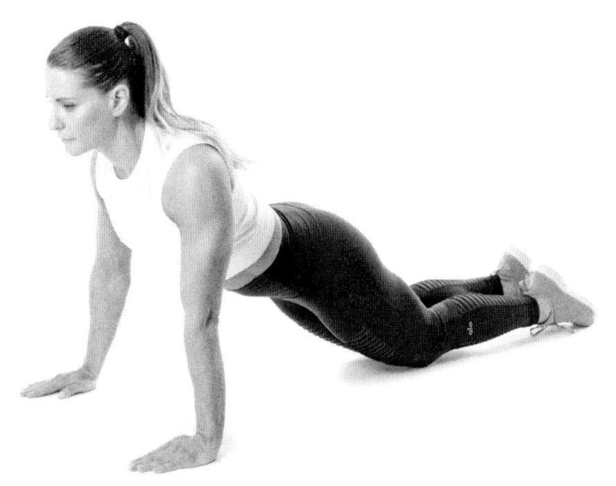

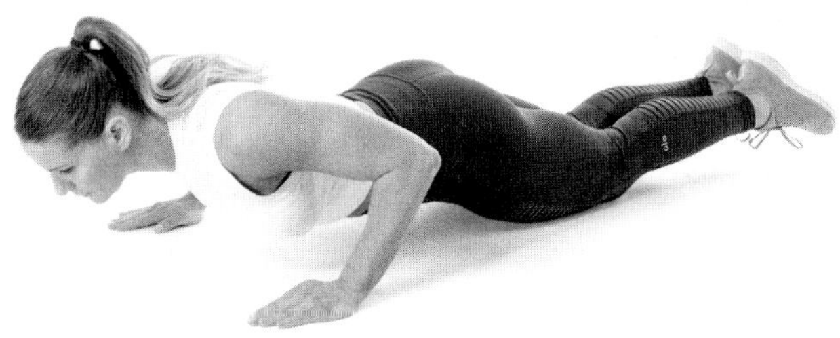

KNEELING CALF STRETCH

Kneel with your right leg bent underneath you and your left leg extended straight in front of you. Reach forward, feeling a gentle stretch in the left calf. Gently pull on the toes of your left foot if you are able.

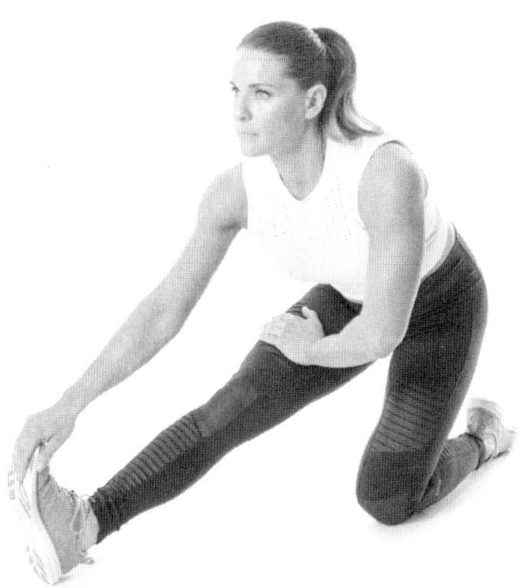

KNEELING HAMSTRING STRETCH

Kneel with your right leg bent underneath you and your left leg extended straight in front of you. Place your hands on your left leg and lean forward from the hips, feeling a gentle stretch behind your left thigh.

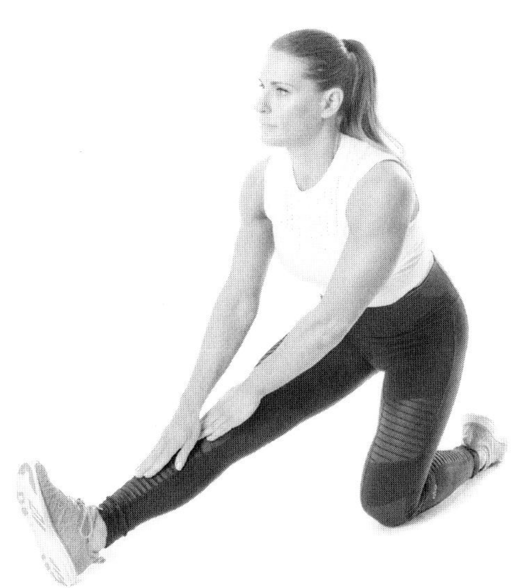

KNEELING HIP FLEXOR STRETCH

Kneel on your left leg with your right leg bent in front of you. Place your hands on your right thigh and slowly push your left hip forward, feeling a gentle stretch in front of the left hip.

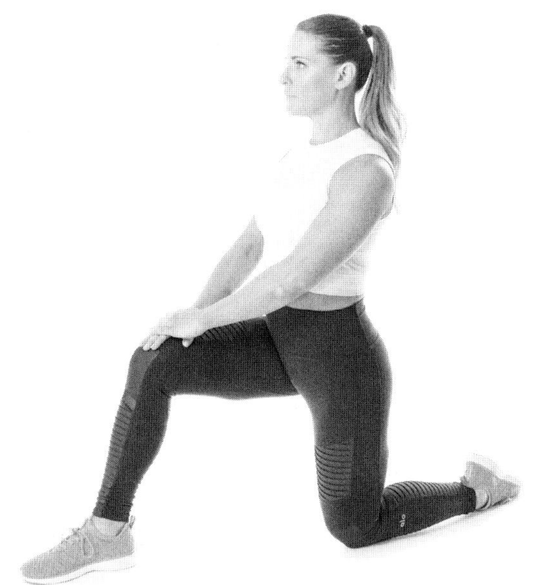

LOW BACK ROTATION

Rotate at the waist to one side, feeling a gentle stretch in the lower back. Hold, then repeat to the other side.

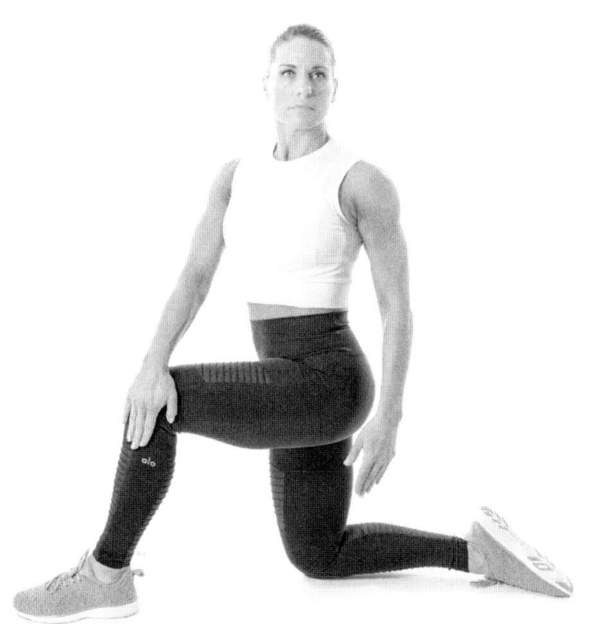

MOUNTAIN CLIMBERS

Assume a push-up position with one leg bent underneath you. Extend the bent leg back while bringing the opposite leg underneath you, alternating quickly back and forth in a running motion.

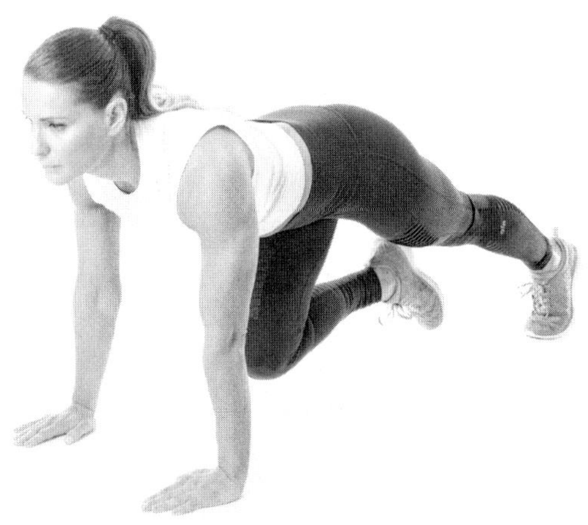

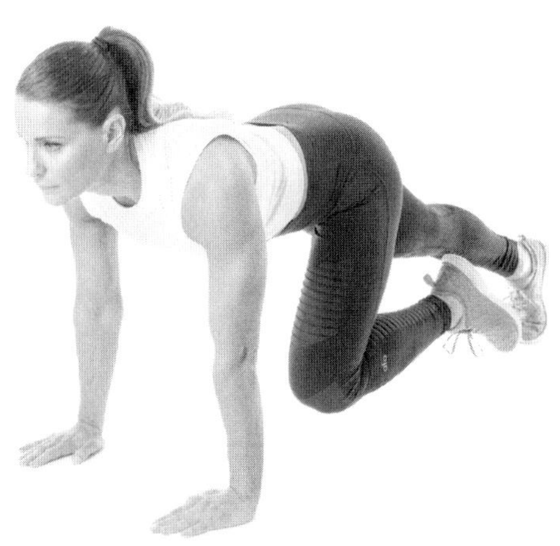

NECK STRETCH

Place your right hand on top of your head. Slowly pull your right ear toward your right shoulder and hold, feeling a gentle stretch in the left side of your neck. Repeat with your left hand to the left side.

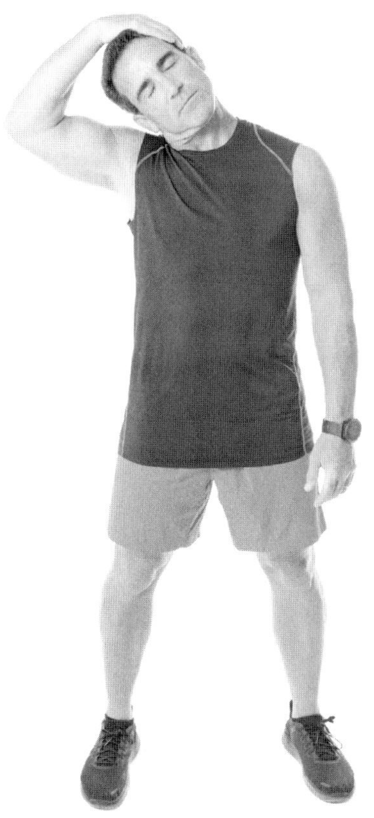

ONE-DUMBBELL OVERHEAD EXTENSIONS

Hold a dumbbell with both hands behind your head. Slow straighten your arms while extending the dumbbell over your head, then return to starting position.

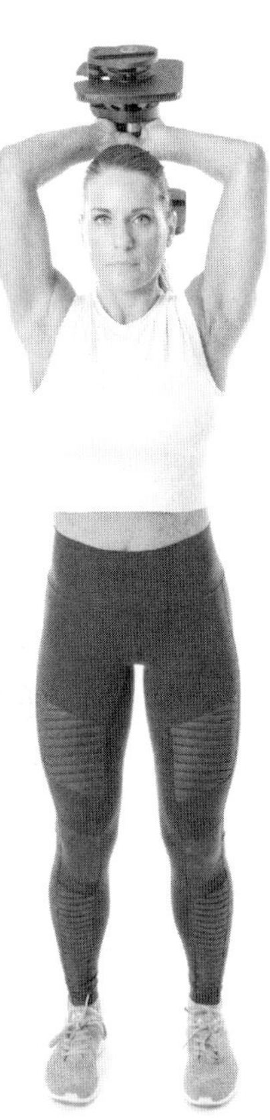

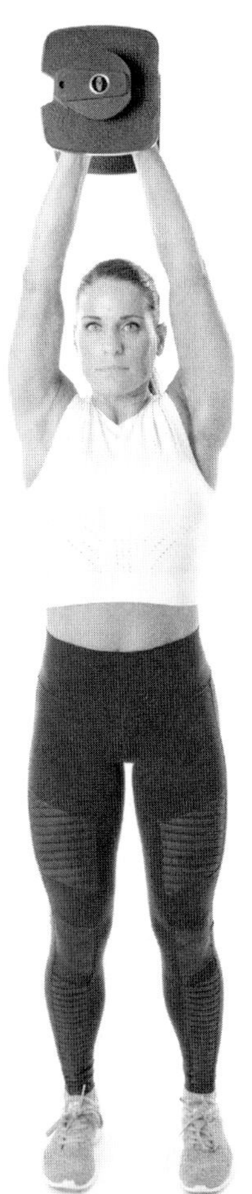

ONE-LEG DUMBBELL DEADLIFT

Stand on one leg with knee slightly bent, holding a dumbbell in the opposite hand. Slowly hinge at the hips and lower the dumbbell toward the floor, keeping the slight bend in the knee and your back perfectly flat, then return to starting position. Do not round the lower back.

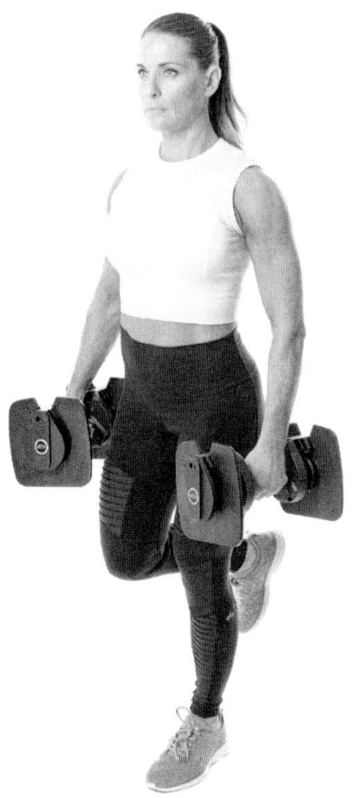

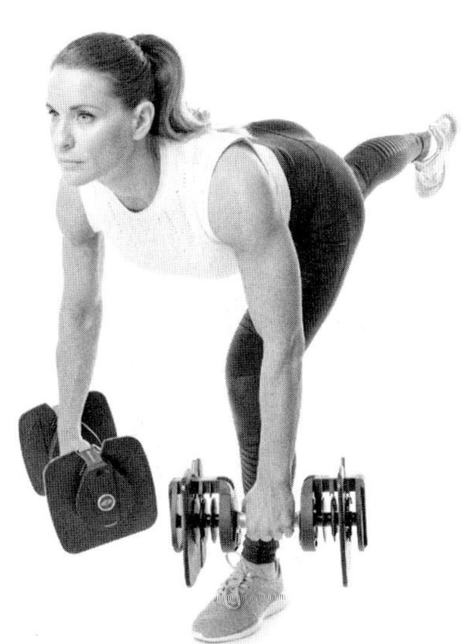

ONE-LEG FLOOR TOUCH

Stand on one leg with knee slightly bent. Slowly hinge at the hips and reach down to the floor with the opposite hand, then return to starting position.

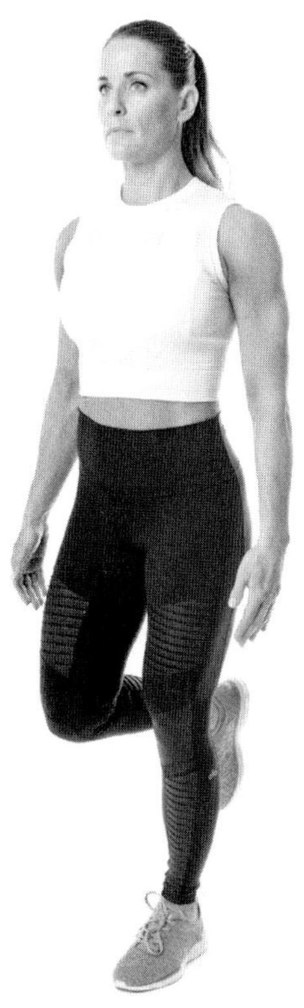

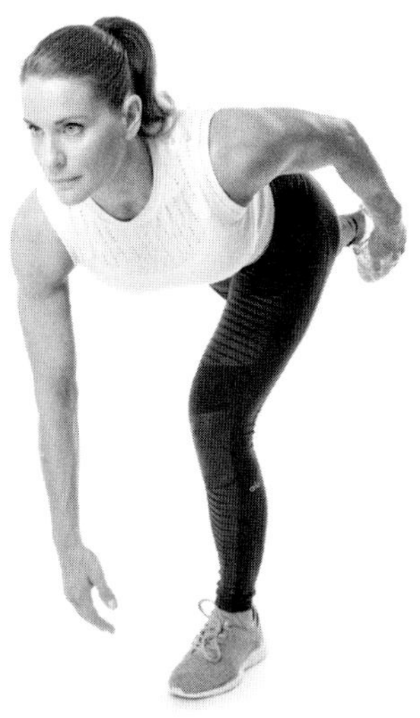

ONE-LEG STAND UP

Sitting on a bench or box with both feet on the floor, stand up using only one leg until the leg is fully extended, then slowly lower yourself back down.

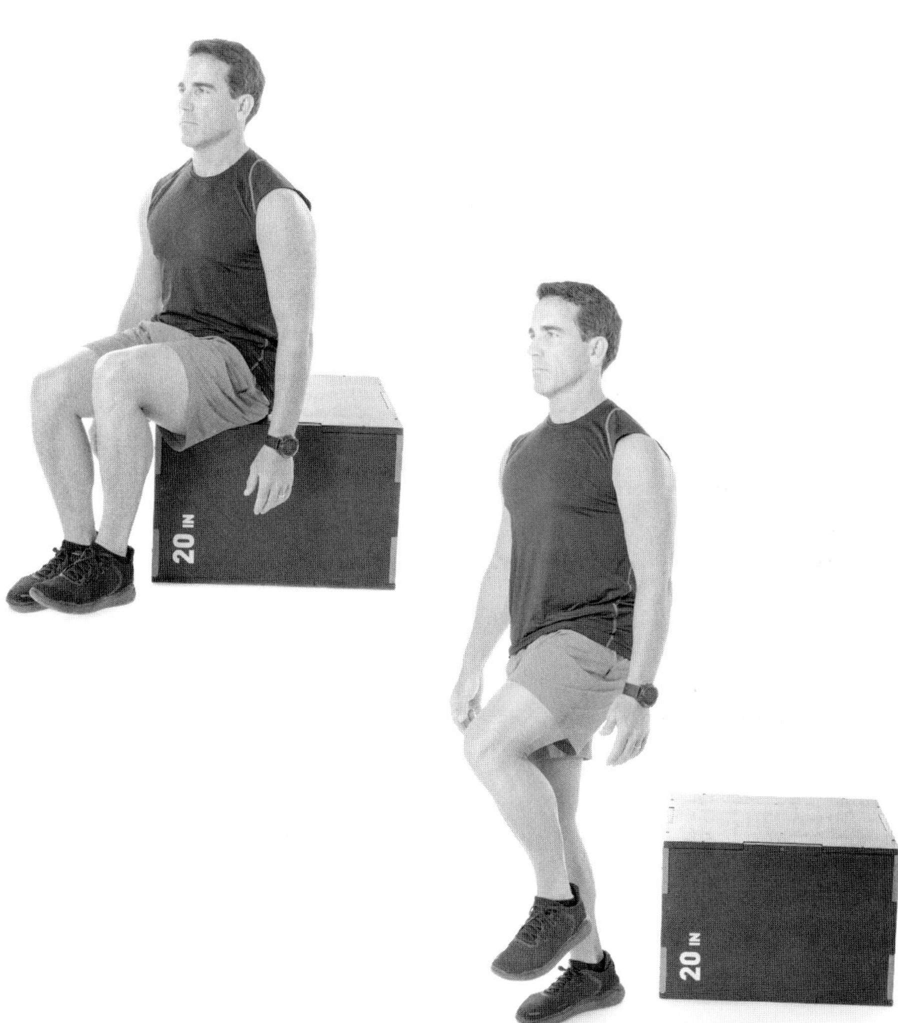

POP SQUATS

Standing with feet shoulder-width apart, jump both feet out to your sides and down into a squat position, and then jump back to starting position.

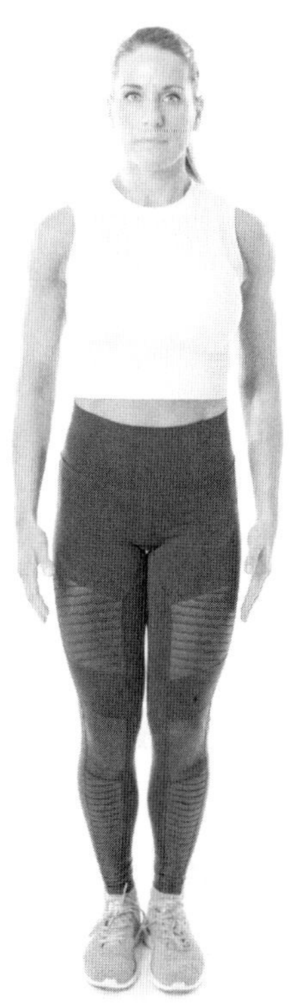

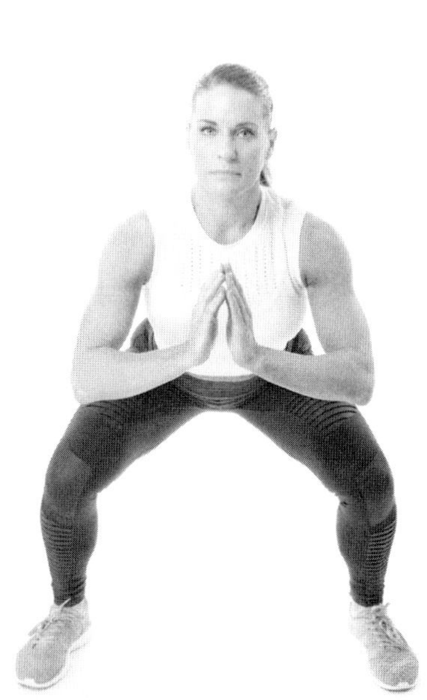

PUSH-UP WITH ALTERNATE RAISED LEG

Hold your body up off the floor with your arms straight and a little wider than shoulder-width apart, your feet a few inches apart, and your body straight and balanced on your hands and toes. Lift one leg off the floor and slowly bend your elbows until your chest is a few inches off the ground, then return to starting position. Alternate legs.

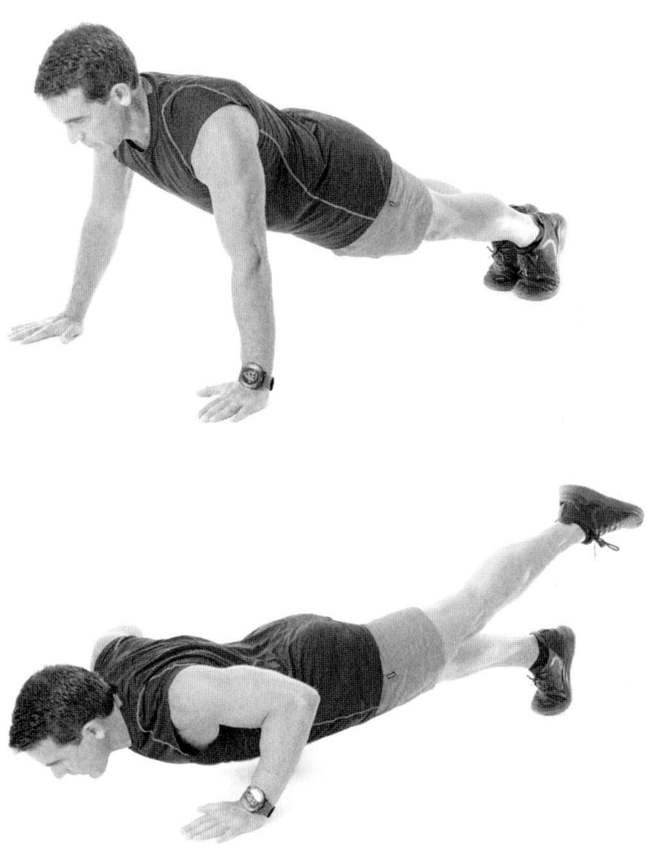

PUSH-UP/ROW COMBO

Grasping dumbbells with your arms straight underneath your shoulders and palms facing each other, hold your body perfectly straight while balanced on the dumbbells and your toes.

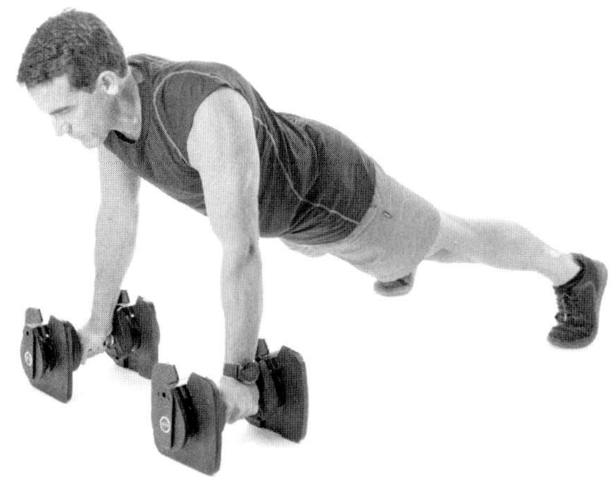

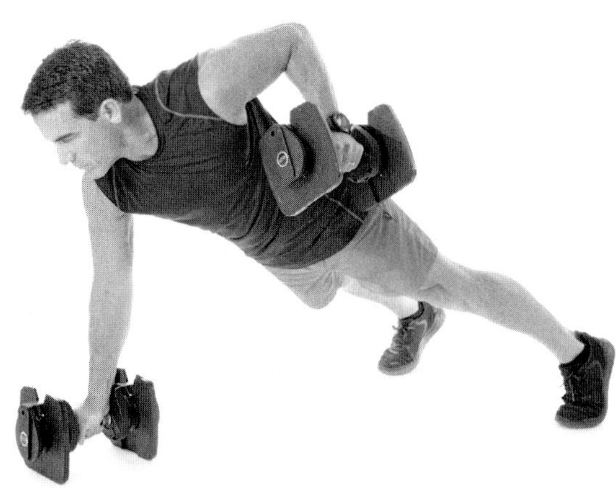

Keeping your body straight, bend your elbows until your chest is a few inches from the floor, then return to starting position. Bring one dumbbell up toward your side and then back down to starting position. Repeat with the other dumbbell.

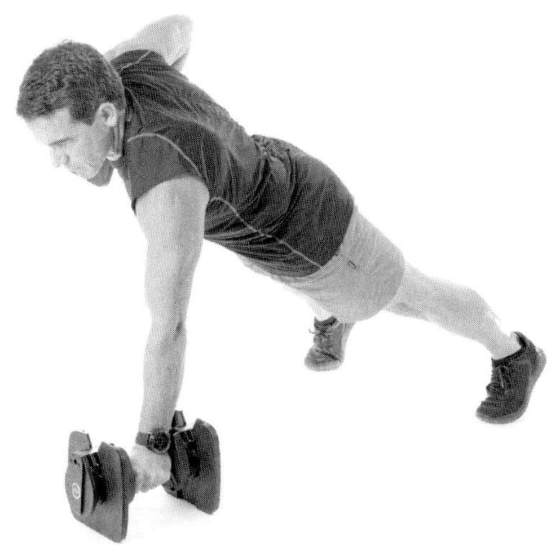

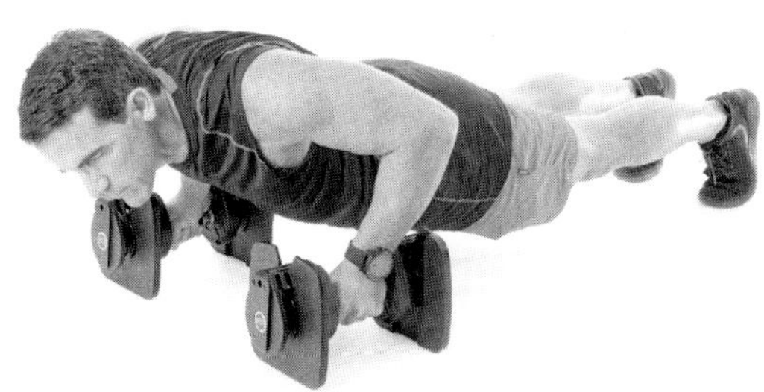

REGULAR CRUNCH

Lie on the floor with your knees bent and your hands behind your head. Keeping your chin off of your chest, slowly lift your upper body off the floor, hold for 1 second, then lower.

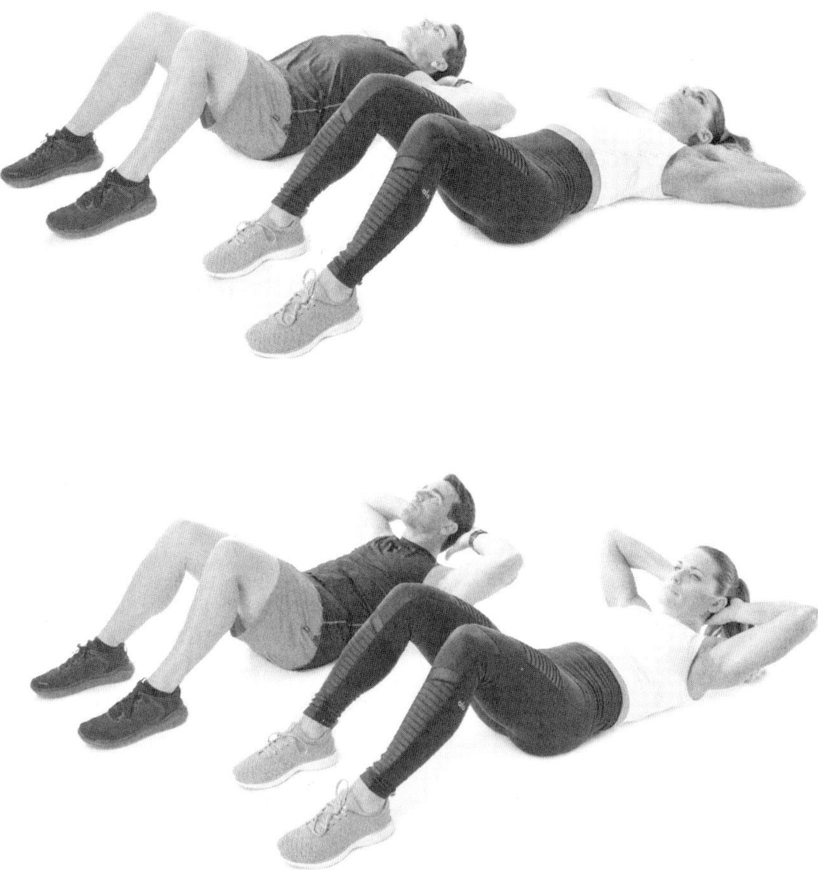

REGULAR PUSH-UP

Holding your body up in a straight line on your hands (just slightly more than shoulder-width apart) and your toes, lower slowly until your chest is a few inches off the floor, then return to the starting position.

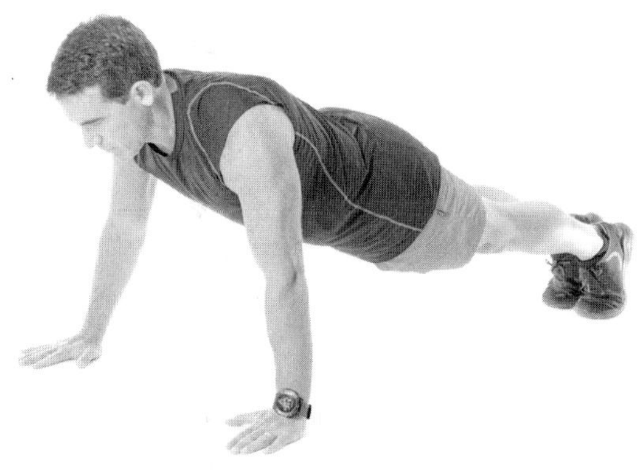

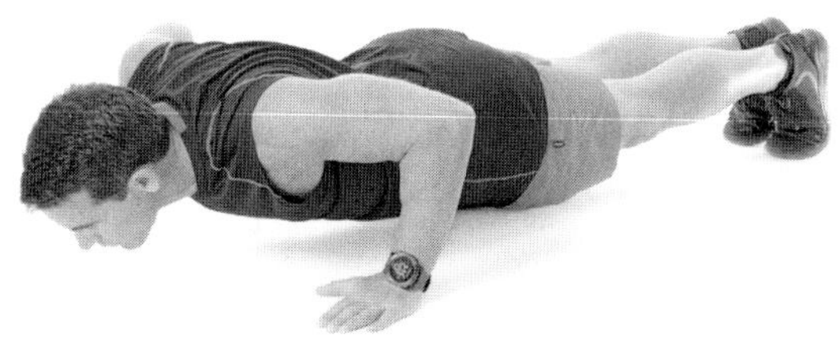

REVERSE CRUNCH

Lie on your back with your legs bent and raised off the floor and your arms at your sides. Pull your knees toward your chest, then return to starting position.

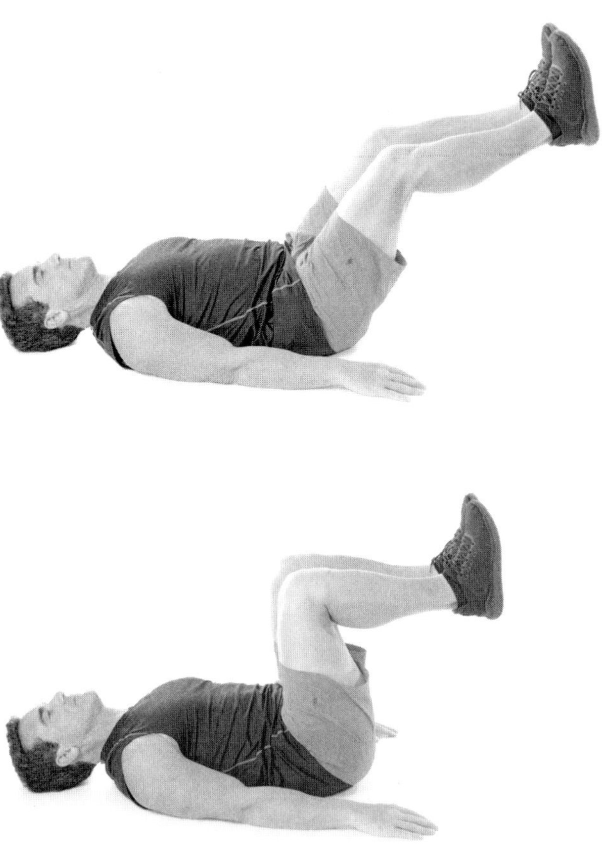

RUNNING IN PLACE

In a standing position, pump your arms back and forth while lifting one foot, then the other.

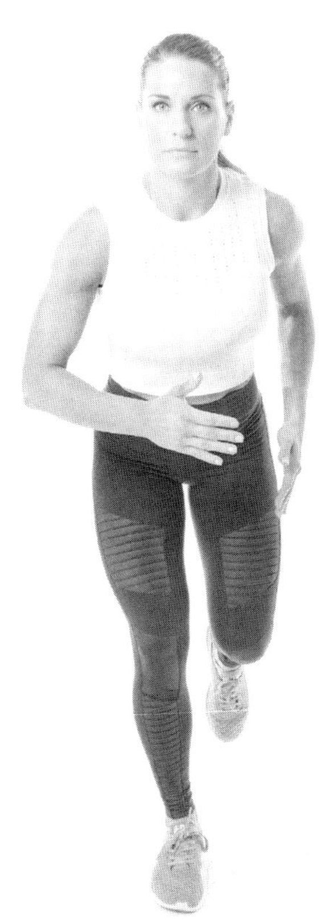

SCARECROW ROTATION

Hold dumbbells with your arms bent 90 degrees and in line with your shoulders, palms facing the floor. Keeping your upper arms still, rotate the dumbbells backward until your palms are facing forward and the weights are directly above your elbows. Hold for one second, then slowly return to starting position.

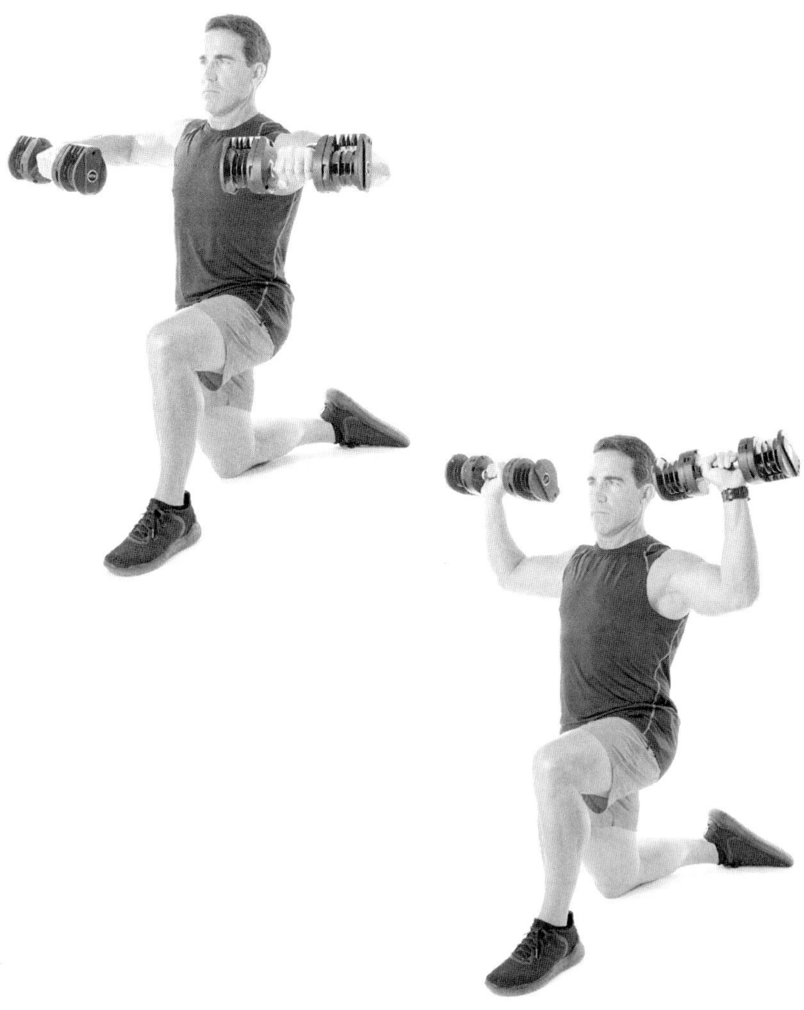

SEAL

Lie on the floor with your hands at your sides. Simultaneously lift your upper body and your feet up off the floor, squeezing the muscles of your lower back and your glutes. Hold for 1 second, then slowly lower.

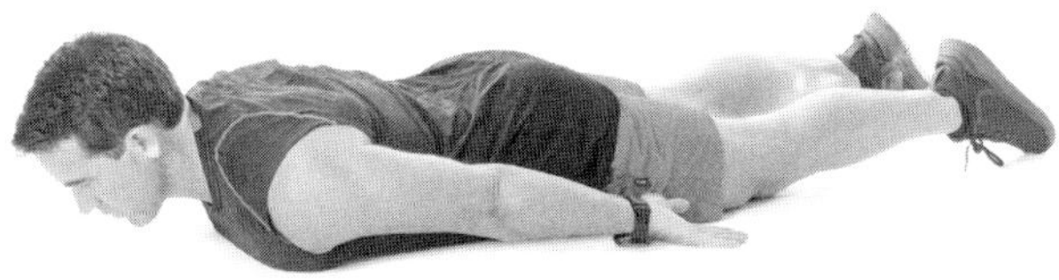

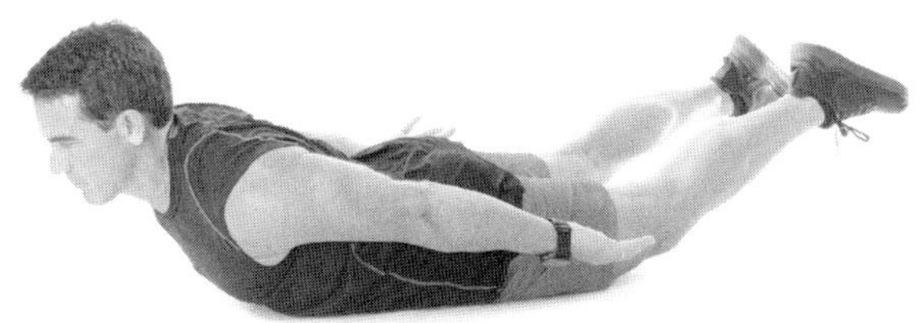

SHOULDER STRETCH

Cross one arm straight across your chest at shoulder height. Gripping your forearm with your opposite hand, gently pull the arm in toward your body, feeling a gentle stretch in your shoulder.

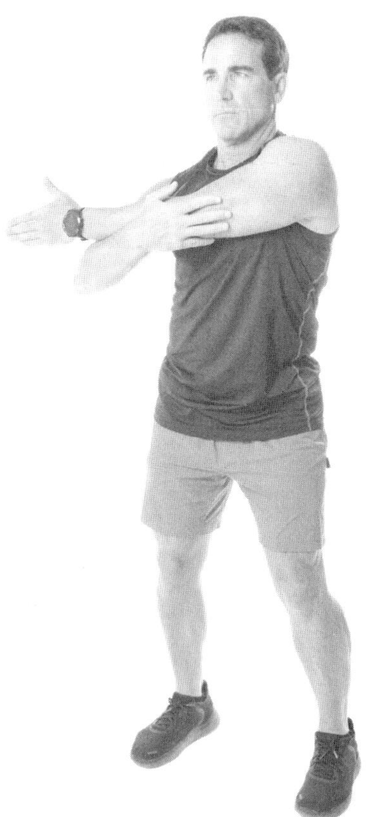

SIDE OBLIQUE CRUNCH

Lie on your left side with your right arm behind your head, your knees bent to 90 degrees, and your left arm on the floor in front of you for balance. Bring your elbow toward your hip, hold for 1 second, then lower and repeat.

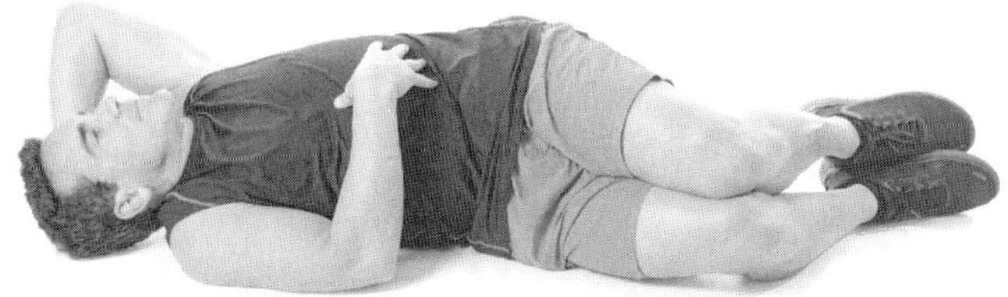

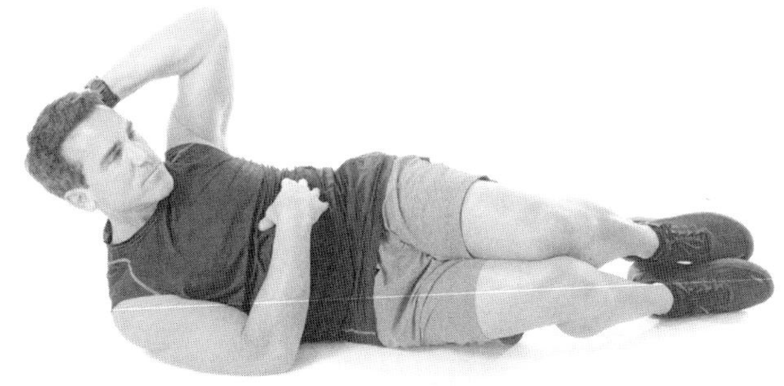

SIDE PLANK

Lie on your side with one arm bent underneath you at 90 degrees and your opposite arm resting on your body. Raise your hips and legs off the ground until your body forms a straight line and hold.

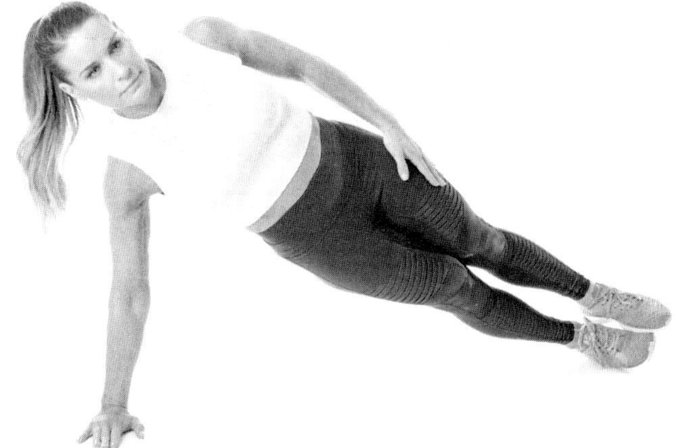

SIDE QUAD STRETCH

Lie on your left side with your hips stacked. Bend your right leg and grab the toes of your right foot, pulling your heel toward your butt while feeling a gentle stretch in the front of your right thigh.

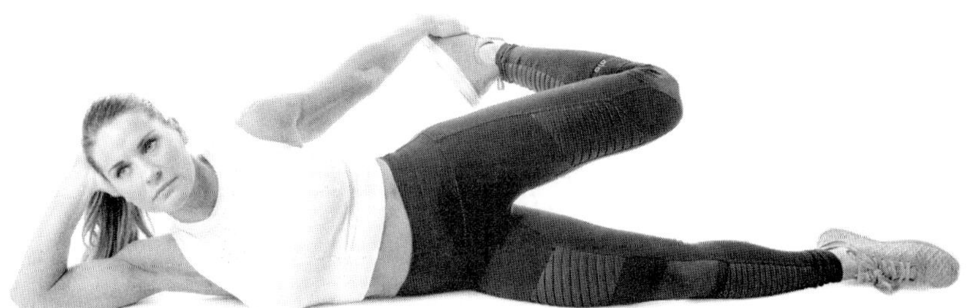

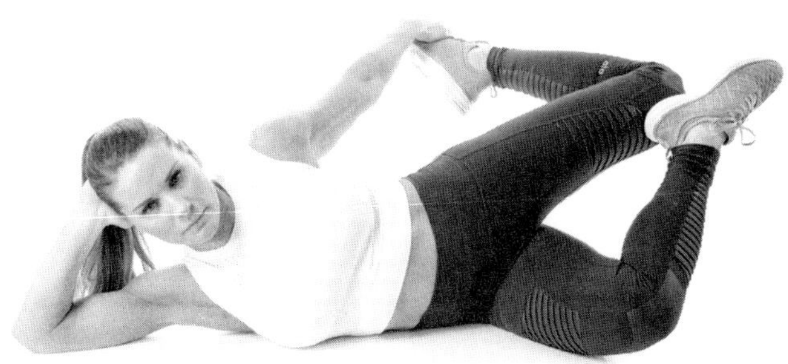

SIDE SCISSORS CRUNCH

Lie on your left side with your right arm behind your head, your knees bent to 90 degrees, and your left arm on the floor in front of you for balance. Bring your elbow toward your hip as you lift your legs off the ground, hold for 1 second, then lower your legs and repeat.

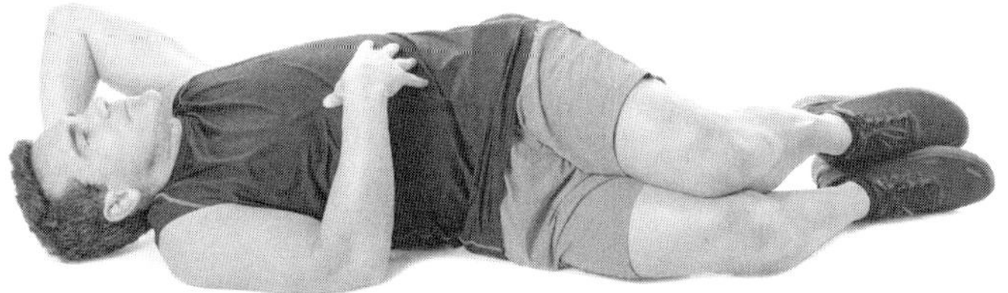

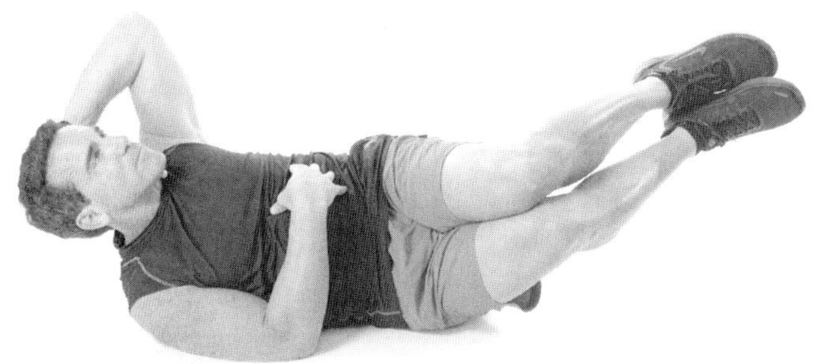

SKATERS

From a standing position, jump to the right and land on your right foot while bringing your left leg behind you, then jump quickly to the left, landing on your left foot with your right leg behind you. Alternate jumping side to side.

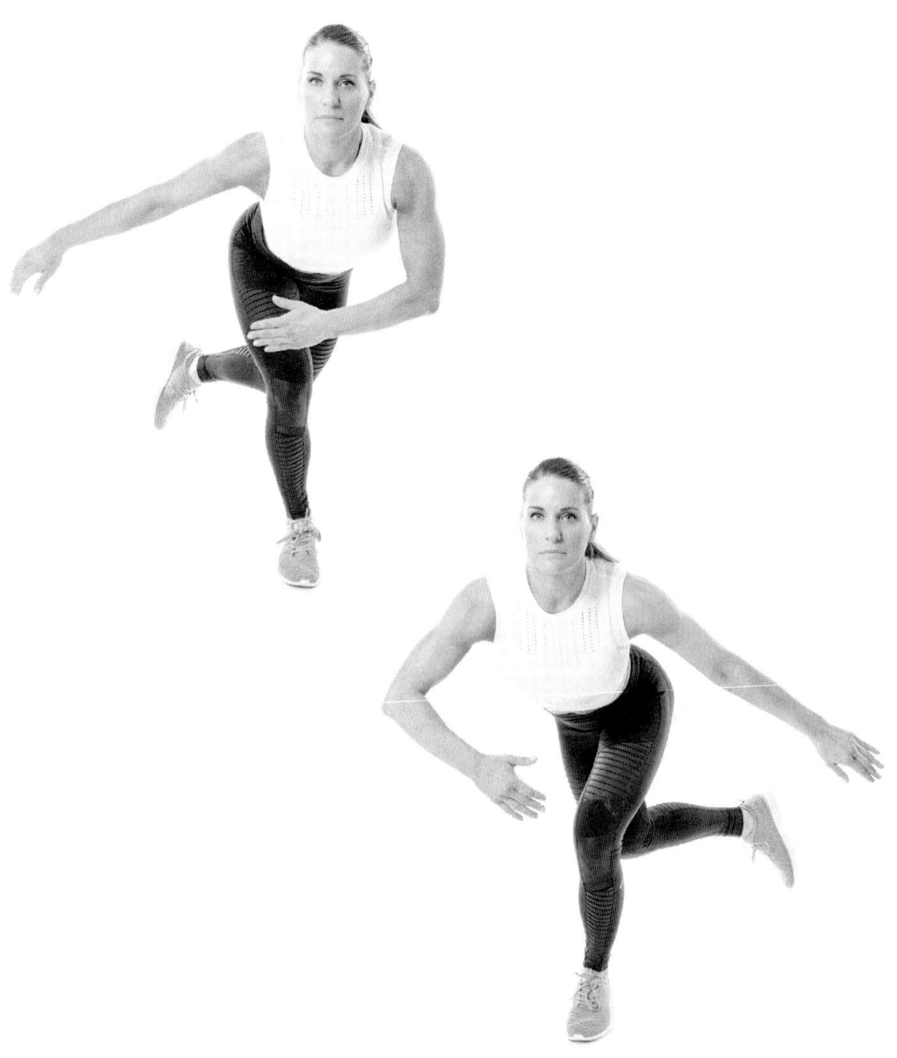

SQUATS

Stand with your feet a little wider than shoulder-width apart and your toes pointing forward, holding a pair of dumbbells at your sides. Keeping your chest up and your knees behind your toes, lower your body until your thighs are parallel to the floor. Hold for 1 second, then return to the starting position.

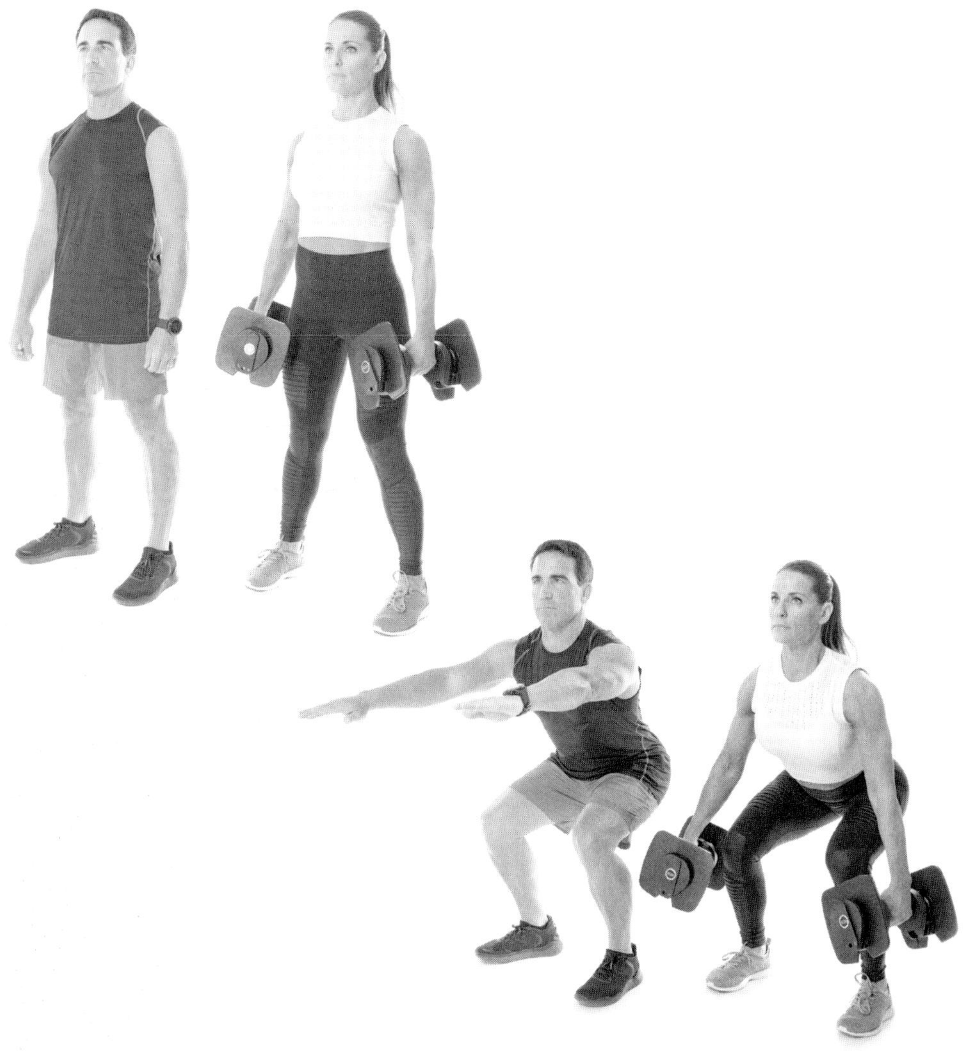

STANDING CALF RAISES

Standing with feet shoulder-width apart, press down on your toes while lifting your heels off the ground as high as you can; hold for one second, then slowly lower back down.

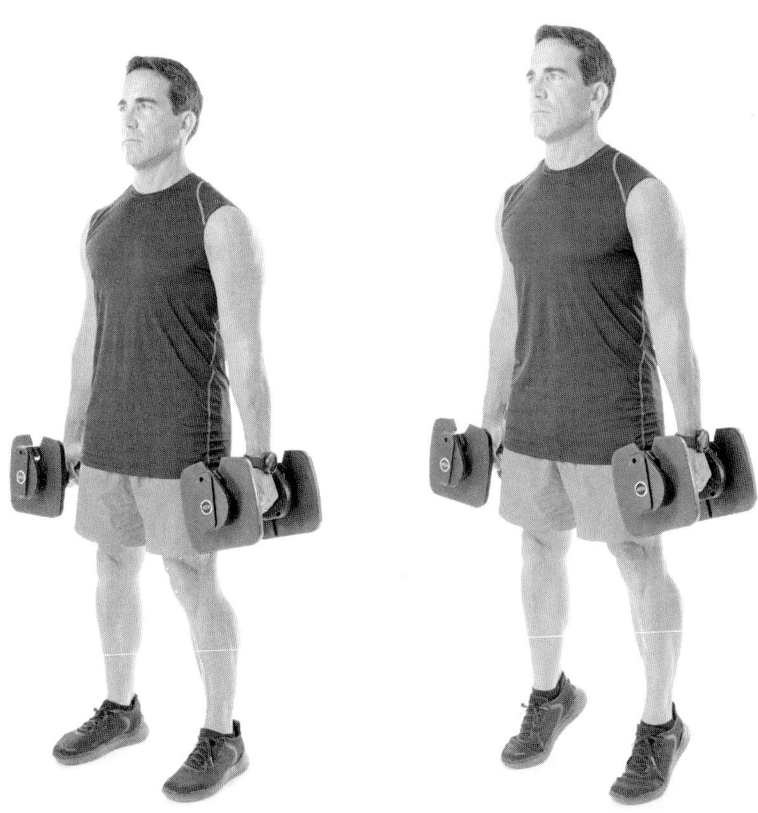

STANDING GLUTE STRETCH

Stand on one leg, cross one ankle above your knee, and slowly sit back into a seated position, feeling a gentle stretch in the glute of the leg that is raised, and hold. You can also hold on to an object such as a chair or bench for support.

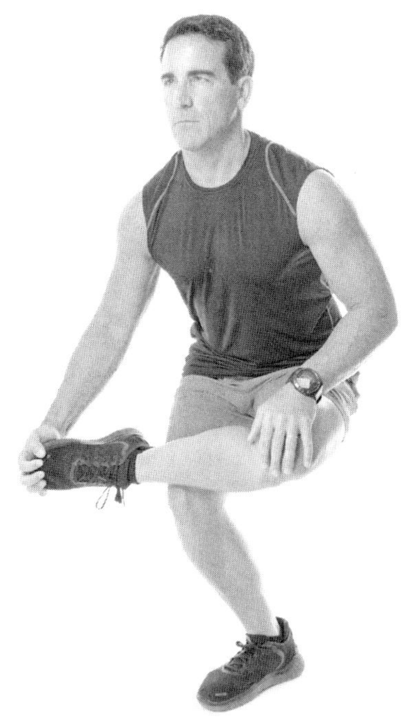

STANDING QUAD STRETCH

Stand on one leg, holding the toes of the other foot while gently pulling your heel toward your butt. Bend your supporting leg slightly and push your hips forward, feeling a gentle stretch in the front of your raised thigh. You can also hold on to an object such as a chair or bench for support.

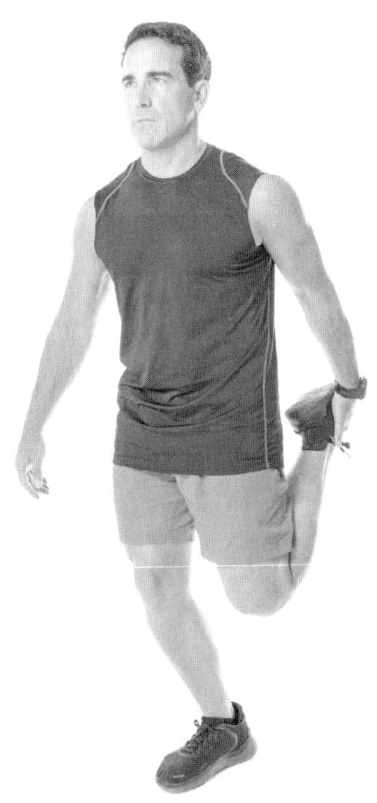

STATIONARY LUNGE

Stand in a split stance with one leg forward and one leg back. Keeping your chest up and your knees behind your toes, lower your body straight to the floor until your back knee is almost touching the floor. Hold for 1 second, then return to the starting position.

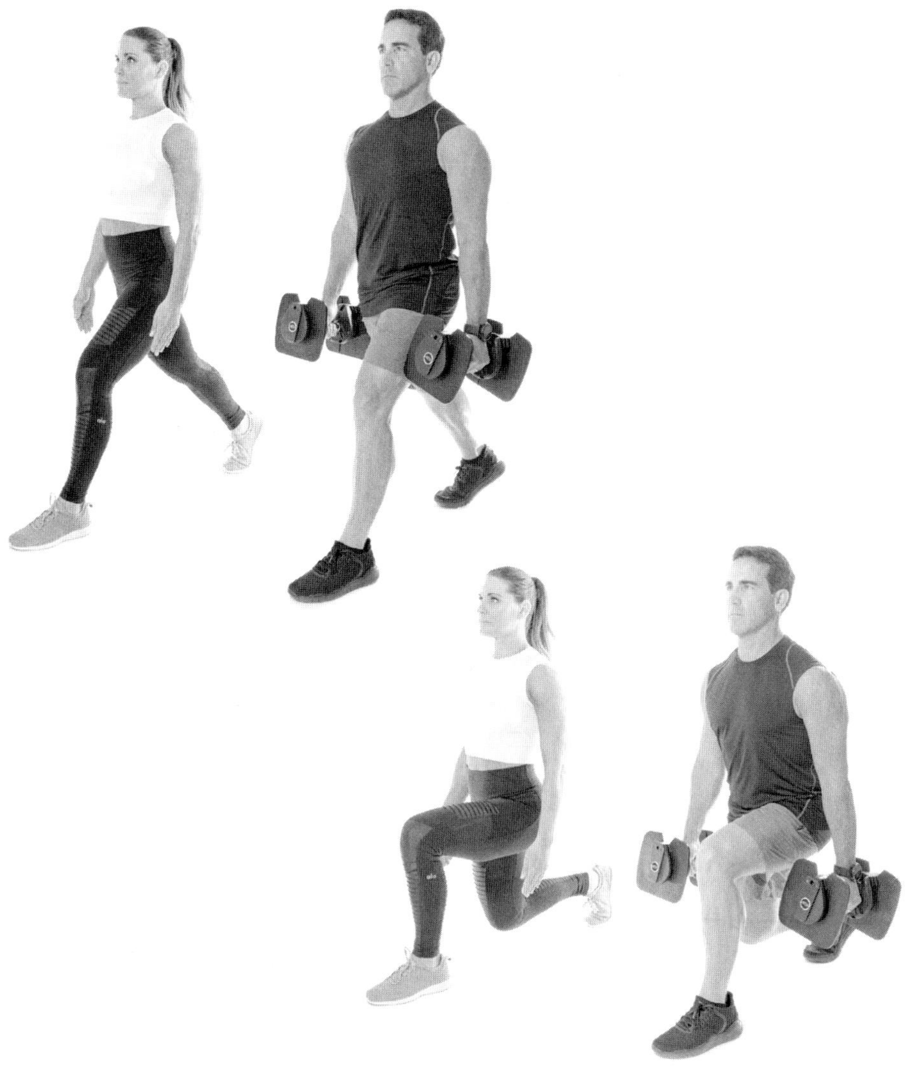

STEP-UPS

Place your right foot on a bench about knee height. Step up and tap your left foot on the bench while fully extending your right leg, slowly step back down with the left leg, then immediately repeat.

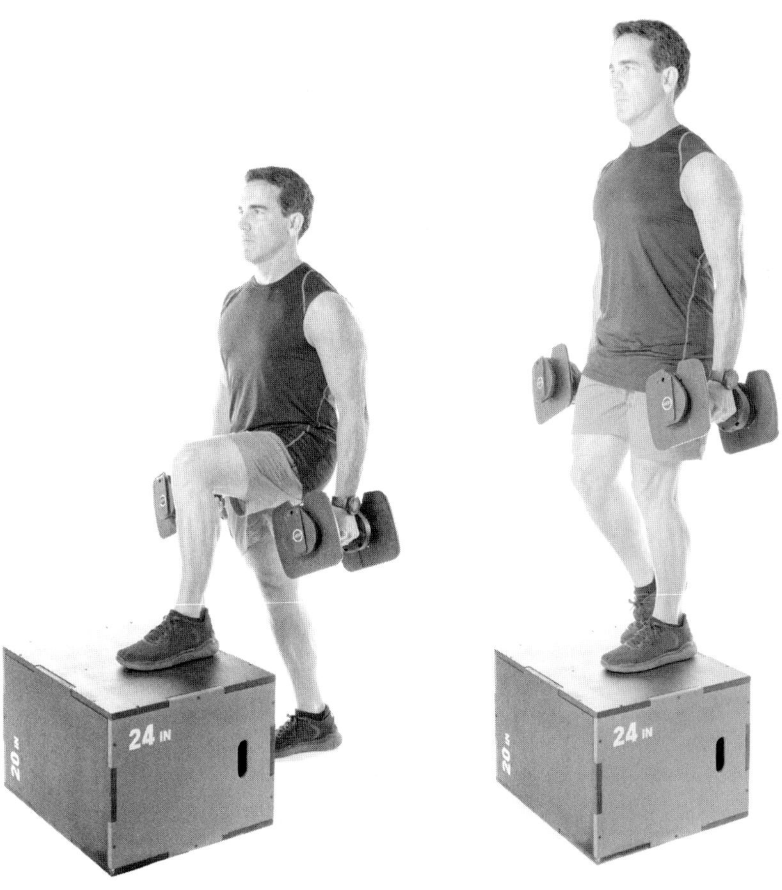

STRAIGHT-ARM PLANK

Assume the top of a push-up position, with your arms fully extended and your body perfectly straight. Keep your body perfectly straight and your abdominals pulled tight, but breathe normally.

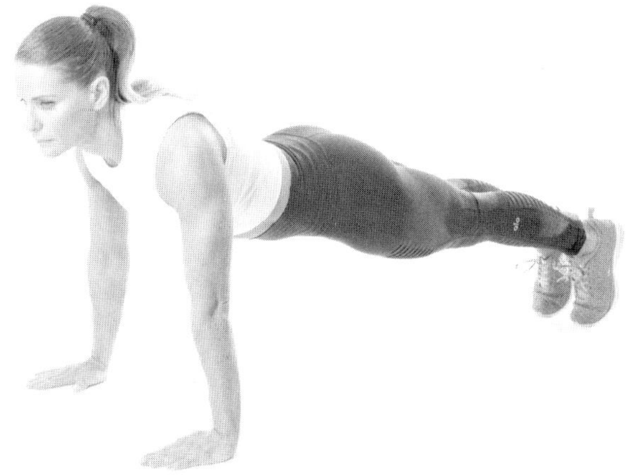

SUPERMAN

Lie on your stomach with your arms straight above your head. Simultaneously lift both hands and feet up off the floor, squeezing the muscles of your lower back and your glutes. Hold for 1 second, then slowly lower.

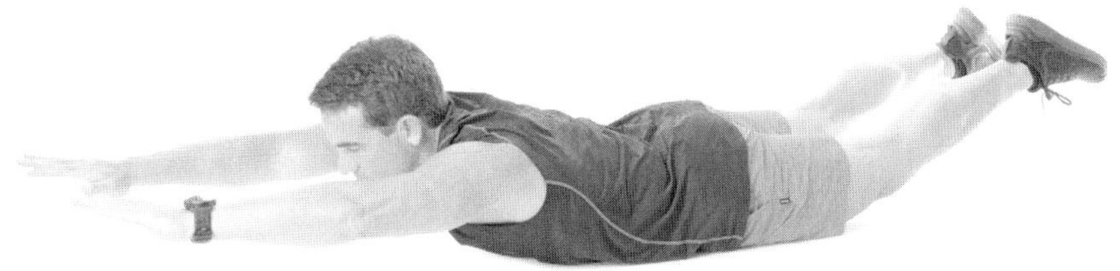

SWIMMER

Lie flat on your stomach with arms straight out on either side of your head. Simultaneously lift your right arm and left foot off the floor, place them down, and repeat with the left arm and right foot.

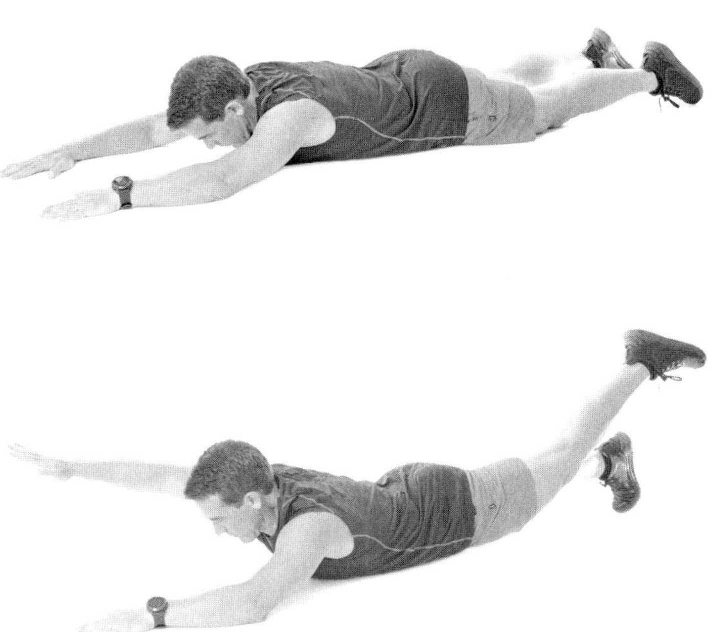

TRICEPS STRETCH

Bend your left arm and bring it behind your head, placing your right hand just behind your elbow. Slowly pull your elbow back while feeling a gentle stretch in the left tricep. Repeat with the other arm.

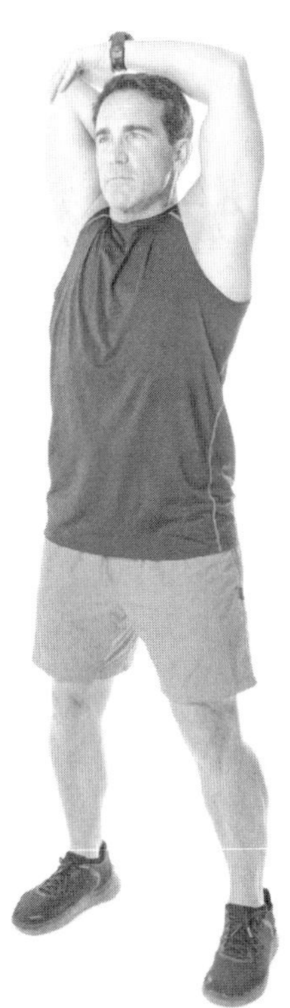

TUCK JUMP

Standing with feet shoulder-width apart, jump up into the air while bringing your knees up toward your chest.

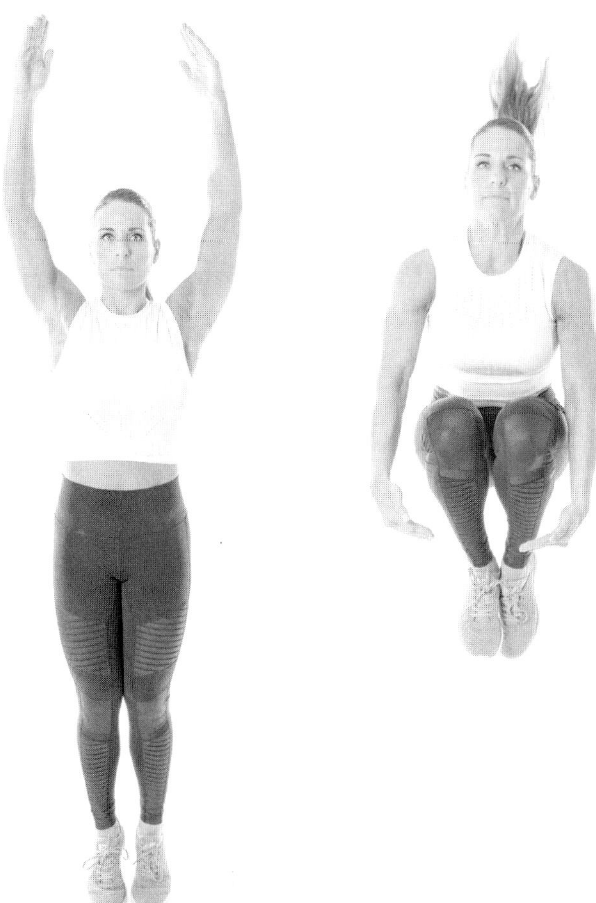

ACKNOWLEDGMENTS

I would like to thank the following people for helping make this book possible: Philippa Holland, John Fread, Aaron Brotherton, Erin Beck, Lori Lasky, Linda Konner, Barbara Berger, Melissa McNeese, Leslie McClure, Sarah Hansson, Andrew Reardon, John Ludwig, Bill and Elissa Oshinsky, Sarah Lavin, The Kahn Family, the Bukovac Family, Michael and Michelle Buscher, Gina Zangrillo, Jim Parsons, the Brannock Family, Drew and Ashley Smith, Billy and Michele Mathews, and Tommy and Cooper Holland.

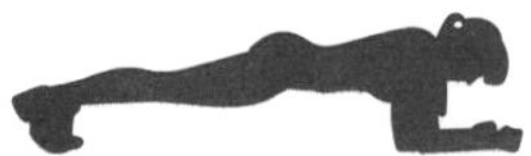

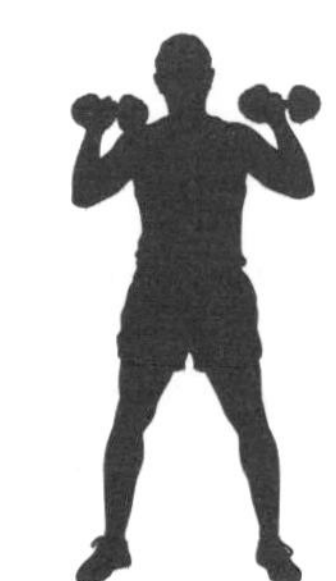

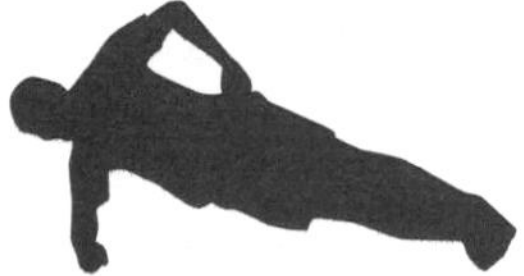

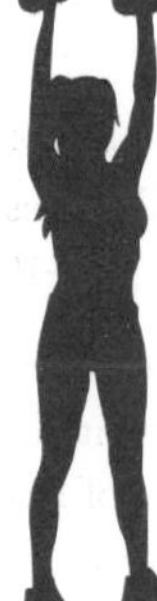

SOURCES

CHAPTER 2 · MYTH-BUSTING

Myth 1: You Can't Escape Your Genetics

Campbell, W. W., M. C. Crim, V. R. Young, and W. J. Evans. "Increased Energy Requirements and Changes in Body Composition with Resistance Training in Older Adults." *American Journal of Clinical Nutrition* 60, no. 2 (August 1994): 167–75, https://doi.org/10.1093/ajcn/60.2.167.

Chodzko-Zajko, Wojtek, David Proctor, Maria Fiatarone Singh, Christopher Minson, Claudio Nigg, George Salem, and James Skinner. "American College of Sports Medicine Position Stand. Exercise and Physical Activity for Older Adults." *Medicine & Science in Sports & Exercise* 41, no. 7 (July 2009): 1510–30, https://doi.org/10.1249/MSS.0b013e3181a0c95c.

Liu, Yanghui, Duck-Chul Lee, Yehua Li, Weicheng Zhu, Riquan Zhang, Xuemei Sui, Carl Lavie, and Steven Blair. "Associations of Resistance Exercise with Cardiovascular Disease Morbidity and Mortality." *Medicine & Science in Sports & Exercise* 51, no. 3 (March 2019): 499–508, https://doi.org/10.1249/MSS.0000000000001822.

Westcott, Wayne. "Resistance Training Is Medicine: Effects of Strength Training on Health." *Current Sports Medicine Reports* 11, no. 4 (July–August 2012): 209–16, https://doi.org/10.1249/JSR.0b013e31825dabb8.

Myth 2: Running Is Bad for Your Knees

Hartmann, Hagen, Klaus Wirth, and Markus Klusemann. "Analysis of the Load on the Knee Joint and Vertebral Column with Changes in Squatting Depth and Weight Load." *Sports Medicine* 43, no. 10 (October 2013): 993–1008, https://doi.org/10.1007/s40279-013-0073-6.

Hinterwimmerm, Stefan, Matthias J. Feucht, Corinna Steinbrech, Heiko Graichen, and Rüdiger von Eisenhart-Rothe. "The Effect of a Six-Month Training Program Followed by a Marathon Run on Knee Joint Cartilage Volume and Thickness in Marathon Beginners."

Knee Surgery, Sports Traumatology, Arthroscopy 22, no. 6 (June 2014): 1353–59, https://doi.org/10.1007/s00167-013-2686-6.

Hyldahl, Robert D., Alyssa Evans, Sunku Kwon, Sarah T. Ridge, Eric Robinson, J. Ty Hopkins, et al. "Running Decreases Knee Intra-Articular Cytokine and Cartilage Oligomeric Matrix Concentrations: A Pilot Study." *European Journal of Applied Physiology* 116, no. 11–12 (December 2016): 2305–14, https://doi.org/10.1007/s00421-016-3474-z.

Lo, Grace H., Jeffrey B. Driban, Andrea M. Kriska, Timothy E. McAlindon, Richard B. Souza, Nancy J. Petersen, Kristi L. Storti, et al. "Is There an Association Between a History of Running and Symptomatic Knee Osteoarthritis? A Cross-Sectional Study from the Osteoarthritis Initiative." *Arthritis Care & Research* 69, no. 2 (February 2017): 183–91, https://doi.org/10.1002/acr.22939.

Miller, Ross. "Joint Loading in Runners Does Not Initiate Knee Osteoarthritis." *Exercise and Sport Sciences Reviews* 45, no. 2 (April 2017): 87–95, https://doi.org/10.1249/JES.0000000000000105.

Williams, Paul T. "Effects of Running and Walking on Osteoarthritis and Hip Replacement Risk." *Medicine & Science in Sports & Exercise* 45, no. 7 (July 2013): 1292–97, https://doi.org/10.1249/MSS.0b013e3182885f26.

Myth 3: You're Too Old to Start

Aagaard, Per, Charlotte Suetta, Paolo Caserotti, Stig Peter Magnusson, and Michael Kjaer. "Role of the Nervous System in Sarcopenia and Muscle Atrophy with Aging: Strength Training as a Countermeasure." *Scandinavian Journal of Medicine and Science in Sports* 20, no. 1 (February 2010): 49–64, https://doi.org/10.1111/j.1600-0838.2009.01084.x.

Hagerman, Fredrick C., Seamus J. Walsh, Robert S. Staron, Robert S. Hikada, Roger M. Gilders, Thomas F. Murray, Kumika Toma, and Kerry E. Ragg. "Effects of High-Intensity Resistance Training on Untrained Older Men. I. Strength, Cardiovascular, and Metabolic Responses." *Journals of Gerontology Series A: Biological Sciences and Medical Sciences* 55, no. 7 (July 2000): B336–46, https://doi.org/10.1093/gerona/55.7.B336.

Henwood, Tim R., and Dennis R. Taaffe. "Improved Physical Performance in Older Adults Undertaking a Short-Term Programme of High-Velocity Resistance Training." *Gerontology* 51, no. 2 (March 2005): 108–15, https://doi.org/10.1159/000082195.

Kekäläinen, Tiia, Katja Kokko, Sarianna Sipilä, and Simon Walker. "Effects of a 9-Month Resistance Training Intervention on Quality of Life, Sense of Coherence, and Depressive Symptoms in Older Adults: Randomized Controlled Trial." *Quality of Life Research* 27, no. 2 (February 2018): 455–65, http://dx.doi.org/10.1007/s11136-017-1733-z.

Latham, Nancy K., and Chiung-ju Liu. "Strength Training in Older Adults: The Benefits for Osteoarthritis." *Clinics in Geriatric Medicine* 26, no. 3 (2010): 445–59, https://doi.org/10.1016/j.cger.2010.03.006.

Liu, Chiung-ju, and Nancy K. Latham. "Progressive Resistance Strength Training for Improving Physical Function in Older Adults." *Cochrane Database of Systematic Reviews* 8, no. 3 (July 2009), https://doi.org/10.1002/14651858.CD002759.pub2.

Melov, Simon, Mark A. Tarnopolsky, Kenneth Beckman, Krysta Felkey, and Alan Hubbard. "Resistance Exercise Reverses Aging in Human Skeletal Muscle." *PLOS ONE* 2, no. 5 (May 2007): e465, https://doi.org/10.1371/journal.pone.0000465.

Schlicht, Jeffrey, David N. Camaione, and Steven V. Owen. "Effect of Intense Strength Training on Standing Balance, Walking Speed, and Sit-to-Stand Performance in Older Adults." *Journals of Gerontology Series A: Biological Sciences and Medical Sciences* 56, no. 5 (May 2001): M281–86, https://doi.org/10.1093/gerona/56.5.M281.

Myth 4: Strength Training Will Make You Bulky

Reynolds, Gretchen. "How Exercise Changes Our DNA." *Well* (blog). *New York Times*, December 17, 2014. https://well.blogs.nytimes.com/2014/12/17/how-exercise-changes-our-dna/.

Srikanthan, Preethi, Tamara B. Horwich, and Chi Hong Tseng. "Relation of Muscle Mass and Fat Mass to Cardiovascular Disease Mortality." *American Journal of Cardiology* 117, no. 8 (April 2016): 1355–60, https://doi.org/10.1016/j.amjcard.2016.01.033.

Myth 6: You Can Spot-Reduce

Ramírez-Campillo, Rodrigo, David Andrade, Christian Campos-Jara, Carlos Henríquez-Olguín, Cristian Alvarez-Lepín, and Mikel Izquierdo. "Regional Fat Changes Induced by Localized Muscle Endurance Resistance Training." *Journal of Strength and Conditioning Research* 27, no. 8 (August 2013): 2219–24, https://doi.org/10.1519/JSC.0b013e31827e8681/.

CHAPTER 3 · THE FIVE COMPONENTS OF FITNESS

Rodriguez, Melissa. "Latest IHRSA Data: Over 6B Visits to 39,570 Gyms in 2018." International Health, Racquet & Sportsclub Association (IHRSA), March 28, 2019, https://www.ihrsa.org/about/media-center/press-releases/latest-ihrsa-data-over-6b-visits-to-39-570-gyms-in-2018/#.

Swift, Damon L., M. Johannsen, Carl J. Lavie, Conrad P. Earnest, and Timothy S. Church. "The Role of Exercise and Physical Activity in Weight Loss and Maintenance Progress in

Cardiovascular Diseases." *Progress in Cardiovascular Diseases* 54, no. 4 (January–February 2014): 441–47, https://doi.org/10.1016/j.pcad.2013.09.012.

Willbond, Stephanie, M. A. Laviolette, Karine Duval, and Etienne Doucet. "Normal Weight Men and Women Overestimate Exercise Energy Expenditure." *Journal of Sports Medicine and Physical Fitness* 50, no. 4 (December 2010): 377–84.

CHAPTER 4 · EXCESSIVE MODERATION

Buch, Assaf, Ofer Kisa, Eli Carmeli, Lital Keinan-Boker, Yitshal Berner, Yael Barer, Gabi Shefer, Yonit Marcus, and Naftali Stern. "Circuit Resistance Training Is an Effective Means to Enhance Muscle Strength in Older and Middle Aged Adults: A Systematic Review and Meta-Analysis." *Ageing Research Reviews* 37 (August 2017): 16–27, https://doi.org/10.1016/j.arr.2017.04.003.

Ibañez, Javier, Mikel Izquierdo, Iñaki Argüelles, Luis Forga, José L. Larrión, Marisol García-Unciti, Fernando Idoate, and Esteban M. Gorostiaga. "Twice-Weekly Progressive Resistance Training Decreases Abdominal Fat and Improves Insulin Sensitivity in Older Men with Type 2 Diabetes." *Diabetes Care* 28, no. 3 (March 2005): 662–67, https://doi.org/10.2337/diacare.28.3.662.

Viana, Valter A. Rocha, Andrea Maculano Esteves, Rita Aurélia Boscolo, Viviane Grassmann, Marcos Gonçalves Santana, Sergio Tufik, and Marco Túlio de Mello. "The Effects of a Session of Resistance Training on Sleep Patterns in the Elderly." *European Journal of Applied Physiology* 112, no. 7 (July 2012): 2403–8, https://doi.org/10.1007/s00421-011-2219-2.

CHAPTER 5 · 60 MINUTES

Department of Health & Human Services USA, Physical Activity Guidelines for Americans, 2nd ed., https://health.gov/paguidelines/second-edition/pdf/Physical_Activity_Guidelines_2nd_edition.pdf.

Ekelund, Ulf, Heather A. Ward, Teresa Norat, Jian'an Luan, Anne M. May, Elisabete Weiderpass, Stephen J. Sharp, et al. "Physical Activity and All-Cause Mortality Across Levels of Overall and Abdominal Adiposity in European Men and Women: the European Prospective Investigation into Cancer and Nutrition Study." *American Journal of Clinical Nutrition* 101, no. 3 (March 2015): 613–21, https://doi.org/10.3945/ajcn.114.100065.

Lean, Michael E. J., Arne Astrup, and Susan B. Roberts. "Making Progress on the Global Crisis of Obesity and Weight Management." *BMJ* 361:k2538 (June 2018), https://doi.org/10.1136/bmj.k2538.

von Loeffelholz, Christian, and Andreas Birkenfel. "The Role of Non-exercise Activity Thermogenesis in Human Obesity," Endotext, www.endotext.org. Updated April 9, 2018. https://www.ncbi.nlm.nih.gov/books/NBK279077/.

CHAPTER 6 · THE POWER OF THE INTERVAL

Klika, Brett, and Chris Jordan. "High-Intensity Interval Training Using Bodyweight: Maximum Results With Minimal Investment." *ACSM's Health & Fitness Journal* 17, no. 3 (May–June 2013): 8–13, https://doi.org/10.1249/FIT.0b013e31828cb1e8.

Viana, Ricardo Borges, João Pedro Araújo Naves, Victor Silveira Coswig, Claudio Andre Barbosa de Lira, James Steele, James Peter Fisher, and Paulo Gentil. "Is Interval Training the Magic Bullet for Fat Loss? A Systematic Review and Meta-analysis Comparing Moderate-Intensity Continuous Training with High-Intensity Interval Training (HIIT)." *British Journal of Sports Medicine* 53, no. 10 (May 2019): 655–64, https://doi.org/10.1136/bjsports-2018-099928.

CHAPTER 9 · THE FOUNTAIN OF YOUTH

Baker, Kristin R., Miriam E Nelson, David T. Felson, Jennifer E. Layne, Renee Sarno, and Ronenn Roubenoff. "The Efficacy of Home Based Progressive Strength Training in Older Adults with Knee Osteoarthritis: A Randomized Controlled Trial." *Journal of Rheumatology* 28, no. 7 (July 2001): 1655–65.

Burton, Louise A., and Deepa Sumukadas. "Optimal Management of Sarcopenia." *Clinical Interventions in Aging* 5 (September 2010): 217–28, https://doi.org/10.2147/CIA.S11473.

Cassilhas, Ricardo C., Valter A. R. Viana, Viviane Grassmann, Ronaldo T. Santos, Ruth F. Santos, Sérgio Tufik, and Marco T. Mello. "The Impact of Resistance Exercise on the Cognitive Function of the Elderly." *Medicine & Science in Sports & Exercise* 39, no. 8 (August 2007): 1401–7, https://doi.org/10.1249/mss.0b013e318060111f.

Devries, Michaela C., Leigh Breen, Mark von Allmen, Maureen Jane MacDonald, Daniel R. Moore, Elizabeth A. Offord, M. Palacios Horcajada, Denis Breuillé, and Stuart M. Phillips. "Low-Load Resistance Training During Step-Reduction Attenuates Declines in Muscle Mass and Strength and Enhances Anabolic Sensitivity in Older Men." Physiological Reports (August 2015), https://doi.org/10.14814/phy2.12493.

Holviala, Jarkko, Janne M. Sallinen, William J. Kraemer, Markku J. Alén, and Keijo Häkkinen. "Effects of Strength Training on Muscle Strength Characteristics, Functional Capabilities, and Balance in Middle-Aged and Older Women." *Journal of Strength and Conditioning Research* 20, no. 2 (May 2006): 336–44.

Lachman, Margie E., Shevaun D. Neupert, Rosanna Bertrand, and Alan M. Jette. "The Effects of Strength Training on Memory in Older Adults." *Journal of Aging and Physical Activity* 14, no. 1 (January 2006): 59–73, https://doi.org/10.1123/japa.14.1.59.

Langoni, Chandra da Silveira, Thais de Lima Resende, Andressa Bombardi Barcellos, Betina Cecchele, Mateus Knob, Tatiane do Silva, Juliana da Rosa, Tamiris de Diogo, Irenio Gomes da Filho, and Carla Helena Schwanke. "Effect of Exercise on Cognition, Conditioning, Muscle Endurance, and Balance in Older Adults with Mild Cognitive Impairment: A Randomized Controlled Trial." Journal of Geriatric Physical Therapy 42, no. 2 (May 2018): 1, https://doi.org/10.1519/JPT.0000000000000191.

Leopold Busse, Alexandre, Wilson Jacob Filho, Regina Miskian Magaldi, Venceslau Antônio Coelho, Antônio César Melo, Rosana Aparecida Betoni, and José Maria Santarém. "Effects of Resistance Training Exercise on Cognitive Performance in Elderly Individuals with Memory Impairment: Results of a Controlled Trial." *Einstein* 6, no. 4 (2008): 402–7.

Martins, Raul Agostinho Simões, Manuel J. Coelho e Silva, Dominika M. Pindus, Steven Cumming, Alves Teixeira, and Monica Verissimo. "Effects of Strength and Aerobic-Based Training on Functional Fitness, Mood and the Relationship between Fitness and Mood in Older Adults." *Journal of Sports Medicine and Physical Fitness* 51, no. 3 (September 2011): 489–96.

Mavros, Yorgi, Shelley Kay, Kylie A. Simpson, Michael K. Baker, Yi Wang, Ren R. Zhao, Jacinda Meiklejohn, et al. "Reductions in C-Reactive Protein in Older Adults with Type 2 Diabetes Are Related to Improvements in Body Composition Following a Randomized Controlled Trial of Resistance Training." *Journal of Cachexia, Sarcopenia and Muscle* 5, no. 2 (June 2014): 111–20, https://doi.org/10.1007/s13539-014-0134-1.

Mayer, Frank, Friederike Scharhag-Rosenberger, Anja Carlsohn, Michael Cassel, Steffen Müller, and Jürgen Scharhag. "The Intensity and Effects of Strength Training in the Elderly." *Deutsches Ärzteblatt* 108, no. 21 (May 2011): 359–64, https://doi.org/10.3238/arztebl.2011.0359.

Tsutsumi, Toshihiko, Brian M. Don, Leonard D. Zaichkowsky, Koji Takenaka, Koichiro Oka, and Taro Ohno. "Comparison of High and Moderate Intensity of Strength Training on Mood and Anxiety in Older Adults." *Perceptual and Motor Skills* 87, no. 3 Pt. 1 (December 1998): 1003–11, https://doi.org/10.2466/pms.1998.87.3.1003.

Yang, Pei-Yu, Ka-Hou Ho, Hsi-Chung Chen, and Meng-Yueh Chien. "Exercise Training Improves Sleep Quality in Middle-Aged and Older Adults with Sleep Problems: A Systematic Review." *Journal of Physiotherapy* 58, no. 3 (September 2012): 157–63, https://doi.org/10.1016/S1836-9553(12)70106-6.

CHAPTER 10 · PREHAB VS. REHAB

Mikesky, Alan E., Steven A. Mazzuca, Kenneth D. Brandt, Susan M. Perkins, Teresa Damush, and Kathleen A. Lane. "Effects of Strength Training on the Incidence and Progression of Knee Osteoarthritis." *Arthritis & Rheumatology* 15, no. 55 (October 2006): 690–99, https://doi.org/10.1002/art.22245.

Unhjem, Runar, Mona Nygård, Lene T. van den Hoven, Simranjit K. Sidhu, Jan Hoff, and Eivind Wang. "Lifelong Strength Training Mitigates the Age-Related Decline in Efferent Drive." *Journal of Applied Physiology* 121, no. 2 (1985): 415–23, https://doi.org/10.1152/japplphysiol.00117.2016.

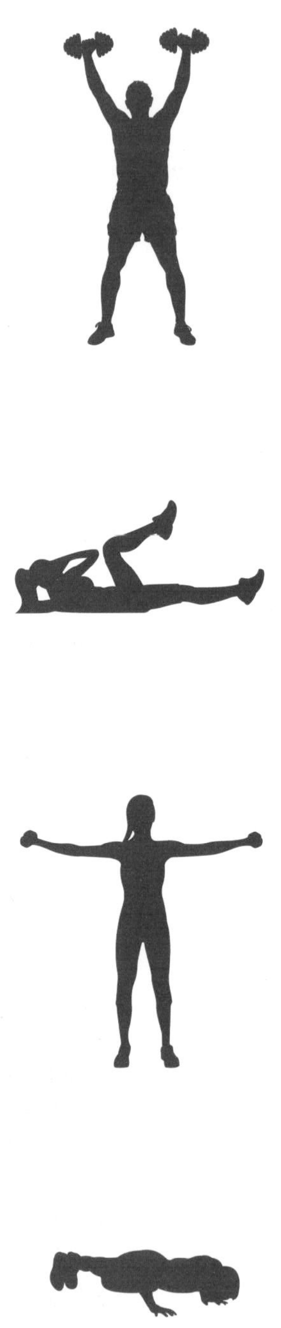

INDEX

Note: Page numbers in *italics* indicate specific exercises.

U

V

W

ABOUT THE AUTHOR AND THE FOREWORD WRITER

TOM HOLLAND is an author, corporate consultant, exercise physiologist, and elite endurance athlete. As the Bowflex® Fitness Advisor, he creates content, markets new products, and hosts weekly fitness videos online. He has served as a celebrity ambassador for Core Hydration, ElliptiGO, FRS Healthy Energy, PowerBar, FitVine, Sportwater, Vega Sports Nutrition, and other companies. He has hosted numerous bestselling fitness DVDs, including *The Abs Diet Workout*, *Supreme 90 Day*, and *Herbalife 24 Fit*, which have sold more than one million copies. He has made more than 100 TV appearances, including on *Anderson Cooper*, *CNN Headline News*, *Good Morning America*, HLN, HSN, QVC, and *Today*. Holland has hosted two national radio shows and appears frequently as a guest on ESPN, SiriusXM, NBC, and Bloomberg Radio, and on the *Wall Street Journal* and Yahoo video channels. He also hosts an iHeartRadio podcast, *Fitness Disrupted*. His fitness advice appears regularly in national newspapers and magazines, including the *New York Times*, the *Los Angeles Times*, *USA Today*, *Men's Health*, *Runner's World*, *Newsweek*, *Cosmopolitan*, and *Prevention*.

Known as "America's favorite fitness expert," **DENISE AUSTIN** has sold over 24 million exercise videos and authored more than twelve books on health and fitness. As a worldwide fitness phenomenon, she has created a loyal audience with her two major television shows: *Getting Fit*, which ran for ten years on ESPN and continued under the new name *Denise Austin's Daily Workout*, and *Fit & Lite*, both on Lifetime.

Denise served two terms on the President's Council on Physical Fitness and Sports. She has testified before the US Senate Committee on Health, Education, Labor, and Pensions; helped launch the new food guidance system of the US Department of Agriculture; and been honored by *Woman's Day* magazine and the American Heart Association with the Red Dress Award for her contributions to heart health.